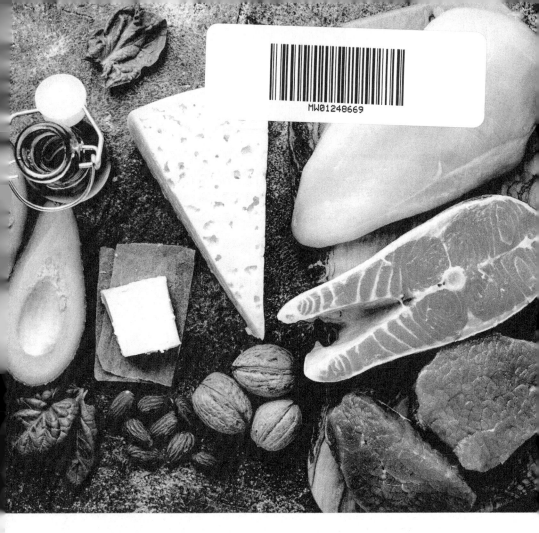

KETO DIET FOR WOMEN OVER 50

COMPLETE GUIDE ON HOW TO PREVENT DIABETES, HAVING A HEALTHY
LIFESTYLE, LOSE WEIGHT, WITH OVER 100 RECIPES!

Liliana Watson

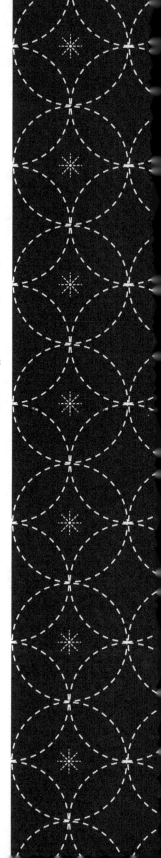

TABLE OF CONTENTS

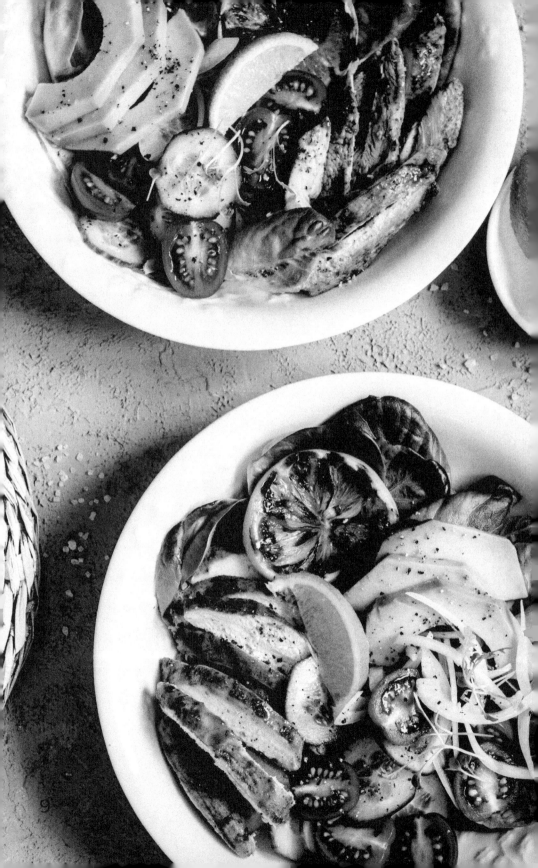

INTRODUCTION

Today's worlds are becoming a more health-conscious and finding way to maintain their healthy weight. Due to the increase in pollution, most of the peoples face a health-related issue like stress, obesity, and hypertension. These health issues are occurring due to unhealthy eating habits.

Keto diet is popular in the 1920s and 1930s used for the therapy of epilepsy. It also used in the treatment of cancer patients; keto prevents cancer cells from using glucose from energy. It starves cancer cells and prevents the growth of cells. Recent research and study prove that the keto diet has used to cure various conditions like Alzheimer's, Parkinson's, epilepsy, metabolic syndrome, obesity, high blood pressure. Keto diet also helps to maintain the blood sugar level in type-2 diabetes patients.

Keto diet is not just a diet it is one of the healthy eating habits and lifestyles. Keto diet is very effective in rapid weight loss. Normally our body uses glucose as a primary source of energy. When you are on the keto diet you consume low carb food. It will reduce the glucose level into your body. Your body burns stored fats for fuel instead of glucose.

This book guides you on how to adopt a keto diet after the age of 50 and what are the health benefits of the diet. The main goal here is to provide you with all related information about keto diet after age 50. After reading this book you should understand what to eat and what to avoid during the ketogenic diet.

CHAPTER 1: WHAT IS DIET?

Starting out on any new diet can be hard, but a ketogenic diet can be one of the hardest to start. This is because it is a sudden change to a completely different way of eating. Carbs are everywhere and we are programmed to eat as many as we can, so most of us have not had a carb-free day in our entire lives. For this reason, regardless of whether we are starting by reducing our carbs, or going cold turkey, the first few days need to be as easy as possible.

Make sure that you have got rid of all your high carb foods. Some people may do this by eating them all over a week leading up to the first day. Others may throw or give the food away to remove temptation. Either way, you need it gone before you start your diet, to remove all the foods that are likely to make you give up. For this reason it is a good idea to ask other people to keep their carby foods away as well, to prepare your own meals, and to refuse invitations to eat out for a while.

Make sure you have all the foods you will want to eat at home. Check out our recipes nearer the end of the book for an idea of what you will want to have. But the priority is a lot of leafy greens, low carb root vegetables, healthy fats, and lean proteins. If you can, try making meals in advance and freezing them in individual tuppers. And make sure to get some low carb, high fat, high protein snacks, like peanut butter, beef jerky, or boiled eggs. That way you can always have something quick to eat when you need it.

When starting out on a ketogenic diet, you will want to begin with foods you already like. Liver, kale, and almond butter are wonderful additions to a ketogenic diet, but eating things you don't like is not the best way to start a long-term diet. Instead, look through the recipe lists for recipes with foods you love, so that you can truly enjoy your diet.

Next, you will want to start on a morning, when you are not going to work. Stress makes us crave carbs more, and eating carbs is what starts the hunger cycle in the first place. So if we start with an empty stomach, running on ketones from the previous night, and we are going to have a relaxed day or two, we will be able to stick it out through the first few days. This massively improves our chances of success, as the first days are the hardest.

When you start a ketogenic diet, you will find many side effects. Most of them are harmless and just part of your body recovering from a lifetime on a high carb diet. Carb cravings are the most common symptom. We have already discussed why these happen, so it is important to remain calm and try and push through. In the next chapter we will offer some solutions for these hunger pangs, but remember that they are at their worst for only a few days, and after that they will be gone.

Indigestion can occur when you first start a ketogenic diet. This is due to a common mistake people make, assuming that this diet is low in all plants. That is not true. On this diet you will eat large amounts of high fibre, low carb plant foods, fatty fruits like avocado, and nuts and seeds. If you do not eat enough fibre you will find that your meals cause reflux, indigestion, and gut cramping. If you are eating plenty of plants but still suffering reflux, indigestion, and gut cramping, consider eliminating dairy from your diet. Sometimes following a ketogenic diet can make an underlying cow milk protein allergy come to the surface. You always would have had this allergy, but it would have been masked by other aspects of your diet.

Finally, if you suffer stomach cramps, diarrhea, or oily, black stools, then you are eating too much fat. How is it possible to eat too much fat on a low carb, high fat diet? The same way it is possible to pour too much water into a glass. When we are following a ketogenic diet we are using fat as fuel. But we can only absorb so much fat in one go, and burn so much fat. When we eat more fat than we can absorb, our bodies just let it pass through us. This is largely harmless, but has the side effect of damaging our gut bacteria, one of the exact things we are trying to fix with out diet. So if you notice these side effects, start reducing your fat intake until your stools return to normal. Besides these symptoms, you should also experience a whole host of beneficial symptoms. Some of the most beneficial symptoms, like an improvement in metabolism, and weight loss, will take longer to happen. But others happen within days. You will find your appetite begins to come under your control. As your insulin spikes and crashes disappear, your body gets used to having a steady supply of energy. This means that rather than feeling hungry every single time your blood sugar drops, and snacking between meals, you are eating a healthy meal and going straight through to the next one without feeling hungry.

You will find that yeast infections and skin conditions improve, or even disappear entirely. This is because your candida is not being fed, so it has nothing to grow from. Candida causes many types of yeast infection, and several types of skin problem, being the root cause of most cases of dandruff, for starters. It also makes other conditions, like eczema, worse, by irritating the skin and growing under and around dead skin cells.

You will find your moods are more even. That "hungry" feeling you get when your blood sugar drops is not normal. It is your body responding to a lack of glucose, trying to get you to eat carbs. At first you may feel the carb-hungry anger more intensely than usual, but after a couple of days your body gets used to not having those constant spikes and crashes in blood sugar. No energy crashes means no cravings, means no eating carbs, means no spikes, means no more crashes. It is vitally important to fight this cycle and restore order, even if you have no intention of following a ketogenic diet for life.

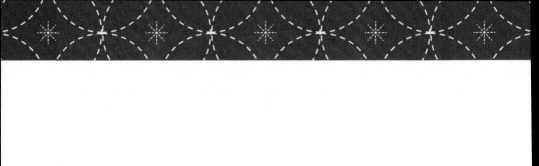

CHAPTER 2: WHAT IS THE KETOGENIC DIET

The ketogenic diet is also known as the low carb diet. It encourages the body to produce ketones from fats in the liver, which are then used by the body as a source of energy in the absence of glucose or sugar.

Glucose is used as a primary source of energy, an excess of it is converted into fats and is stored in many organs such as the liver and adipose tissues. What if you could use up the stored fat as a source of energy and, in doing so, be able to deal with your weight issues? This is where the ketogenic diet comes in.

While it is convenient to fast so that the body can use up most of its fat reserves, not everyone can do fasting. By using and working on the principles of ketosis, the ketogenic diet mimics the metabolic state of ketosis without the hunger.

Look at it this way, if your diet is based primarily on carbs, this then drives the usual metabolic pathway, so you end up storing excess glucose into different parts of the body as fat. Carbs are neither good, nor bad but if you consume too many they can lead to problems like obesity, Type 2 diabetes, and cardiovascular disease.

By eating fewer carbs, you induce your body to the state of ketosis thus making it easier for the body to tap into the stored fat reserves it already has on hand. But getting yourself into the state of ketosis is never easy. Either you go on fasting for days or you cut down your carb intake to 50 grams daily, which is equivalent to around 5% of your total calories.

This can be achieved by changing your diet. Instead of taking in your usual diet, you can drive ketosis by eating more fat and protein. Your fat should be 60-75% of your daily calories while your protein intake should be 15-30% of your calories. This is equivalent to 1 large chicken breast and 5 small avocados each meal. Because fat is naturally filling, it will keep you full for a long time, so you will not feel the need to snack between meals.

The goal for the ketogenic diet is to get your body into the state of ketosis by breaking down fats into ketones as the primary source of fuel by eating the right amounts of food that support such metabolic pathway.

Benefits of Keto Diet Program

Although the ketogenic diet is more called being a speedy fat loss diet regime program', it is truly more to this than meets the eye. The truth is that high rates of energy and weight loss have been still only byproducts of this keto diet, a kind of reward. It has been clinically shown the keto diet program regime has many additional medical benefits.

Let us start with stating that a higher carbohydrate diet regime, together with its lots of ingredients and sugars, has no health advantages. All these are empty calories, and most processed meals fundamentally function to rob your body of those nourishment it needs to stay healthy. Here is a list of real Gains for lowering your carbohydrates and ingestion fats which convert to power:

Control of Blood Sugar

Maintaining blood glucose to a degree that is minimal is critical to avert and to manage diabetes. The keto diet has been proven to be helpful in protecting against diabetes. Many people will also be overweight. That makes an easy regime that a natural. But the keto diet also does more. Carbohydrates have converted into glucose which for diabetics can bring about a sugar spike. An eating plan permits control and low in carbs averts those spikes.

Mental Focus

Even the keto diet is based on protein, fats, and, and low carbohydrates. As we've mentioned, this forces body fat to become the key source of power. This is not the normal diet plan program, that can be conducive to nutrition acids that can be needed for appropriate brain functioning. If folks suffer from cognitive diseases, like Alzheimer's, the mind isn't consuming enough sugar, thus becomes lacking at heart, and the brain has trouble functioning at a higher degree. Increased Energy

It is not Odd, also has become ordinary, to feel drained and tired for a consequence of a poor food plan at the conclusion of the day. Fat is a much more reliable way to obtain energy, leaving you feeling a lot more vitalized than you would on the "sugar" rush.

Keto and Anti-Aging

A number of diseases really are an all organic effect of the aging process. Scientific tests on mice demonstrate brain cell improvement within the keto diet regime program Even though there have been studies done in humans. Studies have demonstrated that a favorable result of the keto diet program. That which we do understand is that a daily diet full of good antioxidants and nutrients, lower in sugar, high in carbs and nutritious carbohydrates, whereas saturated in carbohydrates, enhances our general well-being. It shields us by your toxic compounds of the diet plan. There is also research indicating that with fatty acids such as fuel rather than sugar may slow the process down, possibly. In addition, the act of consuming some energy and ingesting is an issue of wellbeing, since it prevents obesity and its particular negative effects. Scientific studies are constrained. However, considering the positive effects of the ketogenic diet on our health, it is plausible to assume that this daily diet helps us grow old. There are packed with sugars and foods A typical diet plan damaging to warding the indicators of aging.

Keto and Autism

While gluten proteins are most commonly found in wheat, barley, rye and sometimes oat grains and casein in milk and other dairy products, many pre-made products also contain gluten and casein. To correctly implement a keto diet and to hopefully receive the largest benefits of this lifestyle, it is imperative to read all ingredients on labels to ensure that the product you are buying is keto.

Switching to a keto diet can be difficult at first, especially for those who have "picky eaters" in their homes. One key to successfully making the switch is to have patience. Some scientists believe that gluten and casein have an effect on the brain and their removal can resemble something similar to withdrawal. After one to two weeks on a keto diet, many of these symptoms should dissipate.

Some parents with children on a keto diet recommend removing casein products first, followed by gluten products several weeks later. They report that this is an easier transition for their children to make.

Another tip for implementing the keto diet is to slowly introduce substitute products into your child's diet. This allows your child the opportunity to slowly make the switch, as opposed to in one hail swoop.

Once you and your child have achieved 100% keto, remove all gluten and casein products from your home or your child's view. This will decrease the chances of your child seeing their "old favorite treat", wanting it, being denied it, and engaging in negative behaviors (in other words tantrums and meltdowns.)

Take time prior to beginning this diet to consider what improvements that you would like to see. Collect baseline data on the number of words your child is saying, percentage of the time he or she makes eye contact when their name is called, number of tantrums in a day, and so on. Once you have been living a keto lifestyle for at least 8 weeks, recollect data and look for differences. This is an invaluable tool for monitoring the effect that this diet is having on your child.

Be sure to have your child on a good multivitamin. Many foods that your child currently consumes will no longer be part of their diet once they are keto. These foods often contain fortified minerals and vitamins that are essential to your child's growth. These will need to be supplemented once on a keto diet completely.

Give the diet at least six months. Unlike other products, gluten and casein can take up to six months to be completely absent in your child's system. One reason why people don't report results on this diet may be due to this fact.

Keto and Eyesight

Diabetics understand that high blood glucose can cause a higher chance of developing cataracts. Due to the fact, sugar levels are controlled by the keto diet program plan regime, it can help protect against cataracts and maintain eyesight. This has been shown in a Number of studies involving diabetic People

Is the Ketogenic Diet Really for You?

You have to remember that just like all other diet regimens, not everyone can follow a ketogenic diet. So, before you start this regimen, ask yourself if the ketogenic diet is really for you? Below are the things that you should consider to see if the ketogenic diet is for you.

• How long can I follow this diet? The ketogenic diet is not like your usual fad diet only lasting for a few weeks. In order to see results, it will take you months or even a year. So, if you are someone who cannot follow its principles long-term, then this diet is not for you.

• Will the eating plan fit my food preference, budget needs, and culture? If you follow a strict dietary guideline (veganism or vegetarianism) then you might need to tweak the ketogenic diet to fit your preferences. It may difficult, but not impossible. However, if you find it too much of a hassle to tweak the ketogenic meal plan to fit your preference, you might not enjoy this diet at all.

• Do I have medical conditions that will put me at risk? While the ketogenic diet has therapeutic effects to people who suffer from diabetes and cardiovascular diseases, it is not prescribed among people who suffer from kidney-related problems as the presence of protein and fats can be damaging to the kidneys.

The bottom line is that while the ketogenic diet is good for most people, it may not be advisable for some. So, before you ask yourself if this particular diet is for you, make sure that you seek advice from your nutritionist or physician.

CHAPTER 3: WHY I NEED KETOGENIC DIET?

Since the carbohydrate intake for this particular diet is kept at a very low, carbs are practically absent thus the body is pushed to utilize other forms of energy in the form of fat.

In the absence of fat, the liver takes the fatty acids in the body then converts it into ketone bodies. You have to remember that the body just cannot take fat and use it in its raw form. It has to undergo different processes so that it can be utilized effectively by the body. This is the reason why it needs to convert it into ketone form. This process is called ketosis, and this is what the ketogenic diet is all about.

In a nutshell, there are three types of ketone bodies created during the break down of fatty acids and these include (1) acetoacetate, (2) beta-hydroxybutyric acid, and (3) acetone.

There are numerous benefits of the keto diet aside from weight loss and better energy levels.

• Better blood sugar control: The ketogenic diet lowers the blood sugar levels thus making it a great way to manage or even prevent diabetes. The thing is that the body takes a rest from producing insulin thus it can stabilize itself during ketosis.

• Improved mental focus: Several studies suggest that the ketogenic diet can increase health performance. Because this diet does not spike blood sugar levels, the brain is kept in a stable condition. Moreover, the brain simply loves ketones as its primary source of fuel.

• Reduced cravings and hunger pains: Fats are known to be filling, so this particular diet does not only curb your cravings but also reduces hunger pains.

• Better cholesterol and blood pressure levels: This particular diet regimen can improve triglyceride and cholesterol levels in the body. This reduces the risk of developing clogged arteries.

• Clearer skin: Didn't you know that the ketogenic diet can help improve the quality of your skin? Several studies suggest that people who follow the ketogenic diet often experience clearing of their acne and other skin anomalies. The ketogenic diet, aside from pushing ketosis, also drives the immune system into a frenzy thus it can help eliminate inflammation on the skin.

Before you can experience the many benefits of the ketogenic diet, it is important that you eat mostly fat. But how much fat is too much? When I first started, I had this misinformed idea that all I need to do is to eat all the fatty foods that I see. This was easy as pie, I said. And to tell you the truth, I see countless of dieters out there who make the same mistake that I did.

In order to succeed with the ketogenic diet, you don't need to eat a lot of fat. Rather, you need to smartly break down what you eat to 70-80% fat, 20-25% protein, and 5-10% carbohydrates.

You have to remember that the ratio varies depending on different people thus using an online calculator can greatly help! Make sure that you stick by your macros. The problem with most people is that they tend to eat more protein thinking that protein is always equivalent to fat. Well, not quite. Once you consume protein, the protein will be broken down into a process known as gluconeogenesis and it converts protein into carbs. So, you are back to square one.

To ensure that your body is constantly in the state of ketosis, you need to test the ketone levels in your body to know whether your body is still driving under this state or if you reverted back to your usual glucose-feeding metabolism.

There are several ways to test your body for the presence of ketones. Remember that when your body starts to burn off fats as its main energy source, ketones are spilled over into your blood and urine. And it is even present in you breathe! Since ketones are spilled all over the body, you can test either your urine or breath for its presence. You don't need to punch a tiny hole on your skin for blood testing.

CHAPTER 4: WHAT TO DO AND NOT TO DO TO FOLLOW THE KETOGENIC DIET WELL

Top 10 Healthy Foods You Must Eat and Enjoy as A Successful Ketogenic Dieter

Staying in ketosis by eating the right foods is key to healthy weight loss. It is important that you consume more healthy fats than protein to stay in this particular metabolic pathway. I will constantly stress the importance of following the percentage of 5% carbs, 20% protein, and 75% fats. This means that you need to build your meals around low carb vegetables, healthy oils, and moderate protein. Below are the foods that you can consume to drive ketosis.

• Good fats: Remember that not all fats are created equally. While some fats are bad, some are very healthy for the body. You need to consume more good fats in the ketogenic diet. Your options include MCT oil, coconut oil, butter, olive oil, ghee, avocado oil, and other dairy sources like unprocessed cheese, and cream. Another good source of healthy fat is avocado.

• Meat: Choose from a selection of red meats, pork, chicken, turkey, and organ meats. Consume only a matchbox-sized portion for this diet regimen.

• Fatty fish: Fatty fish is a great source of fatty acids like Omega-3s that are precursors to ketones. Source them from trout, sardines, salmon, herring, and mostly cold-water fishes as they have more Omega-3s than other fishes.

• Eggs: Eggs are good sources of healthy fats and proteins.

• Nuts and seeds: Nuts and seeds are staple food items among keto dieters. Have a steady supply of brazil nuts, almond nuts, walnuts, pumpkin seeds, chia seeds, and cashew nuts.

• Vegetables growing above ground: Low carb vegetables in the form of leafy greens, cucumbers, onions, tomatoes, broccoli, cauliflower, and peppers are allowed in this diet. Basically, all vegetables growing above ground (except some squash varieties and tomatoes) are mostly made up of fiber, water, and less sugar.

• Berries: While most fruits are high discouraged while following the ketogenic diet, there are low sugar fruits that you are allowed to eat, and these include blueberries, limes, lemons, apples, and strawberries.

• Sweeteners: Sweeteners sourced from sugar with a high glycemic index is bad for the ketogenic diet. However, allowed sweeteners include stevia, monk fruits, and erythritol.

• Water: Water is the most acceptable beverage in the ketogenic diet because it contains no calories. But if you are not such a big fan of this particular diet, you can always opt for other beverages such as tea, coffee, and red wine (occasionally).

• Bone broth: Bone broth is not only hydrating but it is also chockfull of electrolytes, healthy fats, and nutrients. It is a great beverage to sip on the keto diet. For added fat, add a small dollop of butter to jump start ketosis.

Top 10 Foods You Definitely Must Avoid During Your Ketogenic Journey

The ketogenic diet is not rocket science. While it limits what type of foods that you can consume, it is not really difficult to eliminate certain food groups from your meals. Below are the types of foods that you need to avoid because they don't drive ketosis in the body.

• Sugar of all types: These include honey, maple syrup, white sugar, brown sugar, molasses, and fruit sugars.

• Soda and fruit juice: Soda and fruit juice (yes, even the natural kind) are full of sugar such as glucose and fructose so they can kick you out of ketosis.

• Snacks: Your favorite snacks such as donuts, cookies, cakes, and chocolate bars are strictly prohibited when you are following the ketogenic diet as they are loaded with a lot of sugar and trans-fat.

• Grains: Grains and starches are broken down into glucose thus they should be avoided at all cost. These include rice, oatmeal, rye, barley, wheat, corn, and basically all types of grains imaginable.

• Fruits: Fruits contain high amounts of fructose. Fruits that contain high amounts of sugar include watermelon, bananas, and many others.

• Root vegetables: Root vegetables like sweet potatoes, potatoes, parsnips, and carrots contain high amounts of starch, which can be converted into simple sugar.

• Processed oils: Ketogenic diet advocates the consumption of healthy fats, but it discourages the consumption of processed oils such as vegetable oil, canola oil, corn oil, and soy oil.

• Alcoholic beverages: Alcoholic beverages such as beer are high in sugar thus it is bad for ketosis.

• Beans and legumes: Beans and legumes are high in starch thus it is converted into glucose.

CHAPTER 5: DAILY NEEDS AND BODY CHANGES AFTER 50 YEARS

For women, the biggest hormonal change that happens is menopause. Menopause is a natural part that every woman experiences as a result of their aging process. Once this hormonal shift occurs, women go through three different stages:

1. Perimenopause

Women can start experiencing hormonal changes related to menopause, years before their menopause actually begins. This stage is known as perimenopause, and the average age that women enter this stage is 46, but, of course this depends on many factors and is different for every woman.

During this stage, periods become unpredictable and less frequent, and this last for about 5 year. This stage lasts 6 years and ends one year after the woman's last period.

Estrogen at this stage – Dips irregularly

2. Menopause

Women enter menopause when they are around 51 or 52 years old. You know you are officially in menopause if one years has passed since the last period (if that's not caused by some other medical condition, that is). Although the menopause symptoms such as night sweats and hot flashes, begin in the perimenopause stage, during actual menopause, they are at its peak.

Estrogen at this stage – Drops rapidly, causing noticeable changes such as bone loss and extreme hot flashes

3. Post-Menopause

Post-menopause is the stage that occurs after menopause is considered over, which varies from woman to woman. Typically, post-menopause occurs during women's 50s. And while the menopause stage is officially finished, most of the symptoms will still be there.

Estrogen at this stage – Continues to drop, which causes natural changes in the body. That may cause for women to continue experiencing menopause symptoms (although not so severe) such as hot flashes.

But why does it all happen? To understand the natural changes in your body better, think of the hormones as little messengers that travel through the bloodstream and bring a dose of regulation to chemical and physical functions in our bodies. For women in their 50s, the main culprit for the change in their bodies are the ovaries.

The ovaries produce the hormones that regulate the reproductive system – estrogen and progesterone. The hormones that control these two hormones are the Folicle-Stimulating Hormone (FSL) and the Lutenizing hormone (LH). At this point, we are more concerned with the FSL hormone.

The FSL hormone is the messenger that sends an order of estrogen production and contributes to the release of eggs from the ovaries. When the woman reaches a certain age and enters perimenopause, her ovaries produce a decreased amount of estrogen because the ovaries have fewer eggs than during the reproductive years. But since the FSL messenger doesn't get the memo that the release order shouldn't be sent because there aren't that many eggs, this hormone actually gets increased. Trying to stimulate the production of estrogen, during these years, women have a higher level of the FSH hormone in their blood.

These hormone fluctuations don't only drag unpleasant symptoms with them, but they also have a serious negative effect on other hormones as well:

Insulin

Science has found out that decreased levels of estrogen can promote insulin resistance, and in turn, increase the blood sugar. We all know that insulin is a hormone produced by the pancreas with the purpose of regulating the glucose levels in our blood. When you have insulin resistance, your body is practically immune to the effects of the insulin. When that happens, your cells do not open up for glucose to enter, which leaves the blood sugar endlessly traveling in the bloodstream. The pancreas then keeps producing more and more insulin to keep up with the higher glucose levels, but it is all in vain. The levels of blood sugar are elevated, and your body is resistant to insulin. This may lead to diabetes, weight gain, and many other health issues.

Ghrelin

It is known that during menopause, women experience a significant rise in the ghrelin hormone. The ghrelin hormone is also called the hunger hormone, as it stimulates the appetite and promotes the storage of body fat:

The ghrelin levels are increased □ You feel hungry and trigger the reward center of the brain □ Your desire for food is increased □ The process of digestion speeds up and allow for calories to be absorbed much faster □ The ghrelin in your gut gets released even faster.

Thanks to the rise in their ghrelin levels, women in menopause struggle with weight gain and experience an increase in abdominal fat.

These hormonal changes cause unpleasant symptoms, during, but also after the menopause transition. The decrease of estrogen may be a natural occurrence, but it puts the body through a very challenging phase of adjusting that causes mood swings, hot flashes, fatigue, insomnia, and a number of other fluctuations in the nervous system and brain. There are some natural therapies that can help women cope with these changes, but most women after 50 will tell you that maintaining weight and keeping the overall health balanced is a real struggle. The most effective way to manage the unpleasant age-related symptoms and restore the hormone balance is to rethink your diet and adapt a Ketogenic lifestyle.

Women over 50 – and those that have already been affected by menopause – besides the menopausal symptoms, in general, share three other health issues in common: low stomach acid, low thyroid function, and a sluggish gallbladder.

Low Stomach Acid

As we grow older, our stomach slows down the production of necessary acid, so most women that go through menopause do not have the adequate levels of acid for their stomachs to be functioning normally. This is obviously an important issue that needs to be addressed, but if thinking about starting a Ketogenic diet, low stomach acid should be especially regulated as it plays an essential role in the digestion of protein, as well as eliminating bad microbes.

Thankfully, regulating stomach acid isn't that tricky. Depending on the severity of your condition, you can restore your gut balance without any special supplements. Doctors say that simply squeezing lemon juice or sprinkling apple cider vinegar over your meat and veggies will help you pre-metabolize the food you consume which will aid the process of digestion.

To boost the quality of your digestive juices, make sure to consume more fermented foods such as sauerkraut and kimchi, fermented drinks such as coconut kefir, and up the ginger intake.

Another trick that can help you improve stomach acid is to be mindful about consuming drinks during meals. Keep in mind that drinking plenty of water with meals only dilutes your digestive juices, so make sure to leave the hydration for outside the meals.

Also, make sure to time your protein consumption. It is best to eat the protein-rich foods in the beginning of the meal for better stomach acid support.

If your condition is more severe and these simple strategies don't do you much good, then you should probably take supplements half-way through mealtimes. These supplements should be high in Betaine HCI, but this is best to be discussed with your doctor.

Low Thyroid Function

Thyroid dysfunctions are not a strange occurrence for women and are especially common for older women or those that have already started experiencing the menopause symptoms. Women over 50 often struggle with hypothyroidism (low function) and experience lower vitality, unstable mood, decrease in energy and an increase in weight.

Choosing the Keto lifestyle itself should take care of the problem if your thyroid hormones are not significantly disbalanced. Burning fat for energy and depriving your body of glucose should make women more flexible metabolically and stabilizes their blood sugar, which should, in turn, support a balanced production of the thyroid hormones.

But if you are suffering from hypothyroidism, you shouldn't put all your money on this Keto benefit. If your thyroid hormones are not balanced, then you should also address this issue by making sure to consume the adequate amount of calories. If your body doesn't receive enough calories, it may go to a conservation state and experience a drop in the T3 thyroid hormone.

Those of you who are seriously struggling with hypothyroidism will benefit the most from a Ketogenic diet combined with carb cycling to increase the calorie intake.

Sluggish Gallbladder

Having a sluggish gallbladder may not seem like a particularly serious issue, but it can surely lead to many health-concerning issues. And besides, if you are willing to give the Keto diet a try, then restoring gallbladder health and bile production is a definite must. Why? Because the gallbladder is know to be the reservoir for bile, and bile being a digestive juice that helps the fat emulsion and the creation of fatty acids, you can easily connect the dots and see why it is so important when you are utilizing ketones for energy.

There are a lot of ways in which you can improve the bile production and restore your gallbladder health. Supporting the stomach acid, eating smaller meals, and staying hydrated can all do wonders for your gallbladder.

Consuming foods that are rich in chlorophyll and higher in fiber can also do the trick. Broccoli, kale sprouts, bitter herbs, and fermented foods all support gallbladder health. But perhaps the most successful natural supplement that people with sluggish gallbladder should try is MCT oil.

MCT oil is a natural product that has been refined from coconut oil. It provides a ketone source that is easy-to-digest and readily absorbed so that your liver and overall digestive tract will not have much work to do. This will relieve the stress on the gallbladder and restore its balance.

CHAPTER 6: FOOD LIST FOR A BETTER KETO DIET

As we know that the ketogenic diet is low carb high fat and an adequate amount of protein diet. The following is the food list that allows during the keto diet.

Fats: Fat is necessary during keto diet because near about 75 to 90percent of calories come from fat.

Oils: Instead of processed oil, use oils come from seeds and nuts some keto-friendly oils are coconut oil, butter, avocado oil, MCT oils, lard, extra virgin olive oil, and macadamia oils.

Nuts and seeds: Nuts and seeds are one of the best choices during keto diet because it is high in fat and low in carb. Some keto-friendly nuts and seeds are brazil nuts, pecans, hazelnuts, walnuts, macadamia nuts, pumpkin seeds, flaxseeds, chia seeds, sesame seeds, almonds, and hemp seeds.

Proteins: Adequate amount of proteins (5 to 20 %) are needed during the ketogenic diet.

Meat: Organic and grass-fed meats prefer during the keto diet. Unprocessed meats are low in carb and high in protein. Beef, pork, wild game, veal, and lamb are the best choices for the keto diet.

Poultry: Chicken, Cornish hen, pheasant, quails, duck, turkey, and eggs are the best choices during the keto diet.

Seafood: Salmon, cod, catfish, mahi-mahi, halibut, tuna, trout, octopus, oyster, clams, and shellfish are the best choice during the keto diet.

Dairy: Use high-fat dairy products instead of low fat because the low-fat dairy product contains added sugar. Heavy cream, butter, yogurt, parmesan cheese, cheddar cheese, feta cheese, Colby cheese, mascarpone, Swiss cheese, and mozzarella is the healthy choice during the keto diet.

Carbohydrates: Keto diet is a low carb diet it requires 5 percent of calories from carb intake.

Fruits: Low calories fruits are preferred during the keto diet. Avocado, lemon, blackberries, raspberries, watermelon, and strawberry are the best choices during the keto diet.

Vegetables: Green and leafy vegetables are one of the healthiest choices during keto diet because they are low in carb and high in nutrients. Spinach, chives, asparagus, radicchio, broccoli, cabbage, Brussels sprout, zucchini, celery, chard, bell peppers, olives, etc.

Drinks: During keto diet drink plenty of water to keep your body hydrated. You can also drink plain water, coconut milk, lemon water, almond milk, and low-carb juices.

Condiments: Condiments are used for flavor, you can use low-carb marinara sauce, soy sauce, unsweetened ketchup, yellow mustard all these condiments are no added sugar.

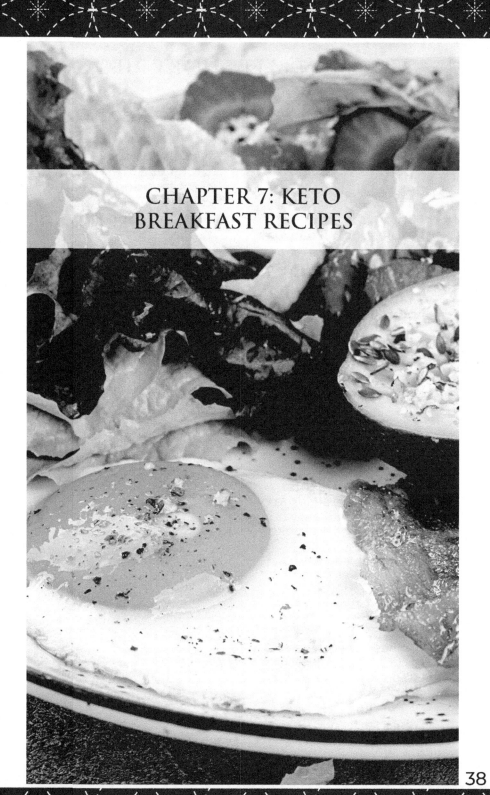

CHAPTER 7: KETO BREAKFAST RECIPES

1. ASIAN BEEF SHORT RIBS

INGREDIENTS

- **2 pounds beef short ribs**
- **1 cup water**
- **1 onion, diced**
- **1 tablespoon Szechuan peppercorns**
- **2 tablespoons curry powder**
- **3 tablespoons coconut aminos**
- **6-pieces star anise**
- **6 tablespoons sesame oil**
- **Salt and pepper to taste**

TOTAL TIME
12 HOURS 20 MINUTES

DIRECTIONS

1. Place all ingredients except for the sesame oil in the Instant Pot.
2. Close the lid and make sure that the steam release valve is set to "Venting."
3. Press the "Slow Cook" button and adjust the cooking time to 12 hours.
4. Once cooked, drizzled with sesame oil.
5. Let it cool. Evenly divide into suggested servings and place in meal prep containers.

Nutrition Information:
Calories 224 kcal — Cholesterol 224mg; — Total Fat 32g — Total Carbs 5g

2. TRADITIONAL FRIED CHICKEN

INGREDIENTS

- **2 large eggs**
- **8 chicken pieces, skin on and bone in**
- **¼ cup heavy cream**
- **¼ cup water**
- **½ cup parmesan cheese**
- **½ tsp onion powder**
- **¾ cup plain whey protein**
- **1 cup crushed pork rinds**
- **1 tbsp oat fiber**
- **1 tsp seasoning**
- **1/8 tsp coarse black pepper**

TOTAL TIME
50 MINUTES

DIRECTIONS

1. Mix all the dry ingredients in a Ziploc bag. Set aside.
2. In a separate bowl, mix together water, eggs and cream.
3. Toss the chicken pieces in the egg mixture.
4. Pick the meat and drop to the bowl of dry ingredients. Toss the bag to evenly coat the chicken. Set aside.
5. Heat a fryer that has ¾-inches of oil in high heat.
6. Place the chicken in the hot oil and cook for 30 to 40 minutes until golden brown.
7. Let it cool. Evenly divide into suggested servings and place in meal prep containers.

Nutrition Information:
Calories 285 kcal — Total Fat 18g — Total Carbs 5.5g — Protein: 6.8g

3. BAKED HERBY SALMON

- **2 pounds salmon fillet**
- **¼ tsp tarragon**
- **¼ tsp thyme**
- **½ cup coconut aminos**
- **½ tsp basil**
- **½ tsp ground ginger**
- **½ tsp rosemary**
- **1 tsp minced garlic**
- **1 tsp dried oregano**
- **4 tsp sesame oil**

TOTAL TIME
20 MINUTES

DIRECTIONS

1. In a Ziploc back, place the sesame oil, soy sauce and spices and shake thoroughly until well combined. Put the salmon pieces in the Ziploc bag. Refrigerate the salmon with the marinade for 4 hours.
2. Preheat the oven to 350oF. Place the marinated salmon on a baking pan lined with aluminum foil.
3. Bake the marinated salmon for 15 minutes.
4. Let it cool. Evenly divide into suggested servings and place in meal prep containers.

Nutrition Information:
Calories per serving: 396; Protein: 47.1g; Fat: 20.9g; Carbohydrates: 1.8g; Fiber: 0.5g

4. CHICKEN COCONUT CURRY

- **1 ½ tsps curry powder**
- **½ onion, sliced**
- **1-lb chicken breast, cut into bite-sized pieces**
- **1 tbsp avocado oil**
- **2 tsps garlic, minced**
- **1 tbsp coconut aminos**
- **1 tbsp ginger, minced**
- **1 ½ cups coconut milk**
- **1/8 tsp salt**

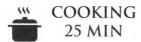 **COOKING** 25 MIN

 **SERVES** 4

DIRECTIONS

1. On medium high heat, place a large nonstick saucepan and heat avocado oil.
2. Add chicken and stir fry for 9 minutes or until chicken is no longer pink. Transfer chicken to a plate leaving oil in pan.
3. Stir fry garlic, ginger, and onion for 3 minutes.
4. Season with curry, coconut aminos, and salt. Sauté for a minute.
5. Return chicken and sauté for 3 minutes.
6. Pour coconut milk, bring to a boil then low heat to a simmer. Simmer for 10 minutes.
7. Let it cool. Evenly divide into suggested servings and place in meal prep containers.

Nutrition Information:
Calories: 257 kcal — Total Fat: 19g — Total Carbs:7.5g — Protein: 11.8g

5. GREEK STYLED LAMB CHOPS

INGREDIENTS

- **1 tbsp black pepper**
- **1 tbsp dried oregano**
- **1 tbsp minced garlic**
- **2 tbsps lemon juice**
- **2 tsp oil**
- **2 tsp salt**
- **8 pcs of lamb loin chops, around 4 oz**

TOTAL TIME
11 MINUTES

DIRECTIONS

1. In a big bowl or dish, combine the black pepper, salt, minced garlic, lemon juice and oregano. Then rub it equally on all sides of the lamb chops.
2. Then place a skillet on high heat. After a minute, coat skillet with the cooking spray and place the lamb chops. Sear lamb chops for a minute on each side.
3. Lower heat to medium, continue cooking lamb chops for 2-3 minutes per side or until desired doneness is reached.
4. Let it cool. Evenly divide into suggested servings and place in meal prep containers.

Nutrition Information:
Calories 104 kcal — Fat 15g — Carbohydrates 4g — Protein 5g

6. ZUCCHINI NOODLES WITH SAUSAGES

INGREDIENTS

- **2 cups of chicken sausages, sliced**
- **2 large zucchinis**
- **2 tablespoons coconut oil**
- **4 garlic cloves, minced**
- **Salt and pepper to taste**

**TOTAL TIME
15 MINUTES**

DIRECTIONS

1. Make the zucchini noodles. You can do this with a mandolin, but you can also slice the zucchini into thin long strips using a knife.
2. In a skillet, heat up the oil over medium heat and sauté the garlic for three minutes while stirring constantly. Add the sausages and cook for another five minutes or until the sausages are cooked through.
3. Add the zucchini and season with salt and pepper to taste.
4. Let it cool. Evenly divide into suggested servings and place in meal prep containers.

Nutrition Information:
Calories 441 kcal — Fat 40g — Carbohydrates 4g — Protein 16g

7. KETO-APPROVED BEEF RAGU

INGREDIENTS

- **1/4-pound ground beef**
- **1 teaspoon salt**
- **2 large zucchinis, cut into noodle strips**
- **1 tablespoon ghee or butter**
- **4 tablespoons fresh parsley, chopped**

TOTAL TIME
15 MINUTES

DIRECTIONS

1. Heat the ghee in a skillet under medium flame and cook the ground beef until thoroughly cooked, around 5 minutes.
2. Add the packaged pesto sauce and season with salt. Add the chopped parsley and cook for three more minutes. Set aside.
3. In the same saucepan, place the zucchini noodles and cook for five minutes. Turn off the heat then add the cooked meat. Mix well.
4. Let it cool. Evenly divide into suggested servings and place in meal prep containers.

Nutrition Information:
Calories 201 — Fat 44g — Carbohydrates 4g — Protein 19g

8. BAKED SALMON WITH LEMON AND THYME

INGREDIENTS

- **1-lb salmon fillet**
- **1 lemon, sliced thinly**
- **1 tablespoon capers, chopped**
- **1 tablespoon fresh thyme, chopped**
- **Olive oil for drizzling**
- **Salt and pepper to taste**

**TOTAL TIME
30 MINUTES**

DIRECTIONS

1. Preheat the oven to 4000F.
2. Line a baking sheet with parchment paper and place the salmon with skin side down.
3. Season the salmon with salt and pepper. Arrange the capers on top of the salmon and top with thyme and lemon slices.
4. Bake for 25 minutes.
5. Let it cool. Evenly divide into suggested servings and place in meal prep containers.

Nutrition Information:
Calories 441 kcal — Fat 64g — Carbohydrates 9g — Protein 23g

9. GARLIC ROASTED SHRIMP WITH ZUCCHINI PASTA

INGREDIENTS

- 8 ounces shrimp, cleaned and deveined
- 1 lemon, zested and juiced
- 2 garlic cloves, minced
- 2 medium-sized zucchini, cut into thin strips or spaghetti noodles
- 2 tablespoon ghee, melted
- 2 tablespoon olive oil
- Salt and pepper to taste

TOTAL TIME
25 MINUTES

DIRECTIONS

1. Preheat the oven to 4000F.
2. In a mixing bowl, mix all ingredients except the zucchini noodles. Toss to coat the shrimp.
3. Bake for 10 minutes until the shrimp turn pink.
4. Add the zucchini pasta then toss. Turn oven off and just leave in oven for 5 minutes.
5. Remove from oven.
6. Let it cool. Evenly divide into suggested servings and place in meal prep containers.

Nutrition Information:
Calories 430 kcal — Fat 19g — Carbohydrates 3g — Protein 21g

10. BACON-WRAPPED ROASTED ASPARAGUS

INGREDIENTS

- **16 asparagus spear, ends trimmed**
- **16 pieces bacon**
- **2 tablespoons extra-virgin olive oil**
- **Salt and pepper to taste**

**TOTAL TIME
15 MINUTES**

DIRECTIONS

1. Preheat the oven to 4000F.
2. Line a baking sheet with aluminum foil or parchment paper. Place the dry asparagus and place it on the baking sheet. Drizzle with olive oil and toss to coat. Add salt and pepper to taste.
3. Wrap each spear with the bacon. Bake for 10 more minutes.
4. Let it cool. Evenly divide into suggested servings and place in meal prep containers.

Nutrition Information:
Calories 632 kcal — Fat 43 — Carbohydrates 15g — Protein 49g

11. SIMPLE COD PICCATA

- **1-pound cod fillets, patted dry**
- **¼ cup capers, drained**
- **½ teaspoon salt**
- **¾ cup chicken stock**
- **1/3 cup almond flour**
- **2 tablespoon fresh parsley, chopped**
- **2 tablespoon grapeseed oil**
- **3 tablespoon extra-virgin oil**
- **3 tablespoon lemon juice**

**TOTAL TIME
20 MINUTES**

DIRECTIONS

1. In a bowl, combine together the almond flour and salt.
2. Dredge the fish in the almond flour to coat. Set aside.
3. Heat a little bit of olive oil to coat a large skillet. Heat the skillet over medium high heat. Add grapeseed oil. Cook the cod for 3 minutes on each side to brown. Remove from the plate and place on a paper towel-lined plate.
4. In a saucepan, mix together the chicken stock, capers and lemon juice. Simmer to reduce the sauce to half. Add the remaining grapeseed oil.
5. Drizzle the fried cod with the sauce and sprinkle with parsley.
6. Let it cool. Evenly divide into suggested servings and place in meal prep containers.

Nutrition Information:
Calories 148 kcal — Fat 15g — Carbohydrates 1.3g — Protein 12g

12. CHICKEN PUTTANESCA

INGREDIENTS

- ¼ cup extra virgin olive oil
- ½ cup assorted Italian olives, pitted and coarsely chopped
- ½ tsp crushed red chili flakes
- 1 lb fresh tomatoes, diced
- 1 small red onion, diced
- 4 boneless chicken breasts
- 4 pieces boneless anchovy filets, coarsely chopped
- 4 pieces garlic cloves, minced
- Pepper and salt to taste

TOTAL TIME
40 MINUTES

DIRECTIONS

1. On high heat, place an oven proof, large skillet.
2. Prepare chicken breasts by seasoning with pepper and salt and greasing with 2 tbsps extra virgin olive oil.
3. Sear chicken on hot skillet around 2 minutes per side or until golden brown on each side. When done searing, lower heat to medium-low, cover and cook until juices run clear. Around 6-8 minutes.
4. Remove from pan and transfer chicken to a platter.
5. On same skillet on medium heat, sauté chili flakes, capers, olives, anchovies, onions, garlic and remaining oil for 2 to 3 minutes.
6. Add tomatoes and season with pepper and salt. Increase heat to high and cook until you have a thick sauce, around 10 to 12 minutes.
7. Pour sauce on top of chicken.
8. Let it cool. Evenly divide into suggested servings and place in meal prep containers.

Nutrition Information:
Calories: 199 kcal — Total Fat: 39g — Total Carbs: 8g — Protein: 15g

13. SUN DRIED TOMATO AND ARTICHOKE CHICKEN

INGREDIENTS

- ¼ cup sun dried tomato pesto
- 1 14.5-oz can diced tomatoes with green peppers and onions
- 1 14-oz can artichoke hearts in water, drained and quartered
- 2 tsps olive oil
- 4 skinless, boneless chicken breast halves
- Pepper and salt to taste

**TOTAL TIME
30 MINUTES**

DIRECTIONS

1. With pepper and salt, season all sides of chicken.
2. On medium high heat, place a large saucepan and heat oil until hot.
3. Add chicken and brown each side, around 5 minutes per side. Once done, transfer chicken to a plate.
4. In same pan, add tomatoes and stir fry for a minute. Scrape all sides of pan to incorporate browned bits.
5. Add artichokes and pesto. Cook and stir for a minute.
6. Return chicken to pan, cover and simmer for 10 minutes on medium heat.
7. Let it cool. Evenly divide into suggested servings and place in meal prep containers.

Nutrition Information:
Calories 550 kcal—Fat 37g — Carbohydrates 06.7g — Protein 24g

14. STEAMED MAHI-MAHI WITH HUMMUS

INGREDIENTS

- **2 filets Mahi Mahi fish**
- **Fresh coriander**
- **2 tbsp lime, squeezed**
- **2 tsp Philadelphia cheese**
- **4 tbsp hummus**
- **Salt and pepper to taste**

TOTAL TIME
35 MINUTES

DIRECTIONS

1. Place Mahi mahi on a heat proof dish that fits in your steamer.
2. Season with pepper, salt, and lime.
3. Sprinkle cilantro on top. Securely cover top of dish with foil and place in steamer.
4. Steam for 30 minutes.
5. Let it cool. Evenly divide into suggested servings and place in meal prep containers.

Nutrition Information:
Calories: 230.9g Fat: 2g; Total Carbohydrate: 32.5 g; Dietary Fiber: 7.0 g; Protein :9.1 g

15. HASHED BRUSSELS SPROUTS

INGREDIENTS

- **4 large eggs**
- **6 slices bacon, cut into 1" pieces**
- **1-lb Brussels sprouts, trimmed and quartered**
- **kosher salt**
- **Freshly ground black pepper**
- **2 tbsp water**

- **2 garlic cloves, minced**
- **1/2 onion, chopped**
- **1/4 tsp red pepper flakes**

TOTAL TIME
50 MINUTES

DIRECTIONS

1. On medium heat, place a nonstick pan and crisp fry bacon. Once done, transfer to a plate and pat away the oil with a paper towel.
2. In same pan with bacon grease, sauté onion for a minute.
3. Stir in Brussels sprouts and cook for 3 minutes.
4. Season with red pepper flakes, pepper, and salt.
5. Add water and continue cooking until liquid has evaporated.

6. Create four holes in the pan and crack eggs. Season eggs with pepper and salt.
7. Cover and continue cooking until eggs are cooked to desired doneness.
8. Let it cool. Evenly divide into suggested servings and place in meal prep containers.

Nutrition Information:
Calories: 50 Fat: 2g; Total Carbohydrate: 10g; Protein :3g

16. STIR-FRIED GROUND BEEF

INGREDIENTS

- **1-lb ground beef**
- **½ cup broccoli, chopped**
- **½ of medium-sized onions, chopped**
- **½ of medium-sized red bell pepper, chopped**
- **1 tbsp cayenne pepper (optional)**
- **1 tbsp Chinese five**

- **spices**
- **1 tbsp coconut oil**
- **2 kale leaves, chopped**
- **5 medium-sized mushrooms, sliced**

TOTAL TIME
20 MINUTES

DIRECTIONS

1. In a skillet, heat the coconut oil over medium high heat.
2. Sauté the onions for one minute and add the vegetables while stirring constantly.
3. Add the ground beef and the spices.
4. Cook for two minutes and reduce the heat to medium.
5. Cover the skillet and continue to cook the beef and vegetables for another 10 minutes.
6. Let it cool. Evenly divide into suggested servings and place in meal prep containers.

Nutrition Information:
Calories: 250; Fat: 10g; carbohydrates: 29g; 2.7 g fiber: 4g; sugar; 2g protein: 4g

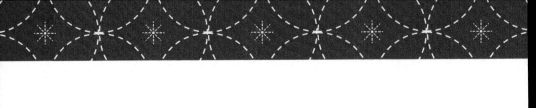

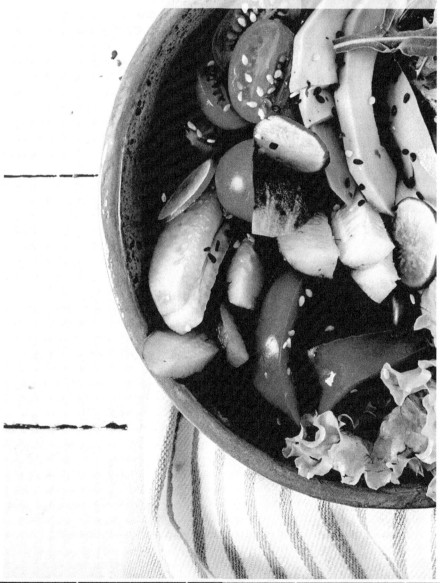

CHAPTER 8: KETO LUNCH & DINNER RECIPES

1. BLUE CHEESE STUFFED PEPPERS

INGREDIENTS

- **4 bell peppers**
- **6 ounces cottage cheese**
- **6 ounces blue cheese, crumbled**
- **½ cup pork rinds, crushed**
- **2 cloves garlic, smashed**
- **1 ½ cups pureed**
- **tomatoes**
- **1 tsp dried basil**
- **Salt and black pepper, to taste**
- **½ tsp chili pepper**

TOTAL TIME
45 MINUTES

DIRECTIONS

1. Briefly boil the peppers for 5 minutes in salted water. Set oven to 360°F.
2. Using a cooking spray, lightly grease the sides and bottom of a casserole dish. In a bowl, mix garlic, cottage cheese, pork rinds, and blue cheese. Stuff the peppers and remove to the casserole dish.
3. Combine the tomatoes with oregano, salt, cayenne pepper, black pepper, and basil. Scatter the tomato mixture over stuffed peppers; use a foil to cover the dish. Bake for 40 minutes until the peppers are tender and serve warm.

Nutrition Information:
Calories 212 kcal — Fat 20.3g — Carbohydrates 5g — Protein 19g

2. QUATRO FORMAGGIO PIZZA

INGREDIENTS

- 1 tbsp olive oil
- ½ cup cheddar cheese, shredded
- 1 ¼ cups mozzarella cheese, shredded
- ½ cup mascarpone cheese
- ½ cup blue cheese
- 2 tbsp sour cream
- 2 garlic cloves, chopped
- 1 red bell pepper, sliced
- 1 green bell pepper, sliced
- 10 cherry tomatoes, halved
- 1 tsp oregano
- Salt and black pepper, to taste

TOTAL TIME
15 MINUTES

DIRECTIONS

1. Set a pan over medium heat and warm olive oil.
2. Spread the bottom with cheddar cheese and cook for 5 minutes until cooked through.
3. Scatter garlic and sour cream over the crust.
4. Add in tomatoes and bell peppers; cook for 2 more minutes.
5. Sprinkle with pepper, salt and oregano and serve while warm.

Nutrition Information:
Carbs: 78; Calories: 369; Total Fat: 0.5g; Protein: 11g;

3. CAULI MAC AND CHEESE

- **1 head cauliflower, cut into florets**
- **2 tbsp ghee, melted**
- **Salt and black pepper, to taste**
- **½ cup crème fraiche**
- **½ cup half-and-half**
- **1 cup cream cheese**
- **½ tsp turmeric powder**
- **1 tsp garlic paste**
- **½ tsp onion flakes**

**TOTAL TIME
15 MINUTES**

DIRECTIONS

1. Set oven to 450°F. Grease a baking sheet with cooking spray.
2. Shake cauliflower florets with melted ghee, salt, and pepper. Arrange on the baking sheet and roast for 15 minutes. In a saucepan over medium heat, pour the remaining ingredients and heat through, stirring frequently. Reduce heat to low and simmer for 2-3 minutes until thickened.
3. Coat the cauliflower florets in the cheese sauce and serve immediately in serving bowls.

Nutrition Information:
Carbs: 10.6; Calories: 211; Total Fat: 3.3g; Protein: 28.1g;

4. CHEESE & PUMPKIN CHICKEN MEATBALLS

INGREDIENTS

- **1 egg, beaten**
- **1 pound ground chicken**
- **1 carrot, grated**
- **2 garlic cloves, minced**
- **1 onion, chopped**
- **1 tbsp Italian mixed herbs**
- **Salt and black pepper, to taste**
- **2 tbsp olive oil**
- **1 cup cheddar cheese, shredded**

TOTAL TIME
35 MINUTES

DIRECTIONS

1. Set oven to 360°F. Combine all ingredients excluding cheese. Form meatballs from the mixture; set them on a parchment-lined baking sheet. Bake for 25 minutes, flipping once.
2. Spread cheese over the balls and bake for 7 more minutes or until all cheese melts.

Nutrition Information:
Calories: 592 kcal— Total Fat: 53g — Total Carbs: 19g— Protein: 33g

5. CHICKEN MEATLOAF CUPS WITH PANCETTA

INGREDIENTS

- **2 tbsp onion, chopped**
- **1 tsp garlic, minced**
- **1 pound ground chicken**
- **2 ounces cooked pancetta, chopped**
- **1 egg, beaten**
- **1 tsp mustard**
- **Salt and black pepper, to taste**

- **½ tsp crushed red pepper flakes**
- **1 tsp dried basil**
- **½ tsp dried oregano**
- **4 ounces cheddar cheese, cubed**

 **TOTAL TIME
0 MINUTES**

DIRECTIONS

1. In a mixing bowl, mix mustard, onion, ground turkey, egg, bacon, and garlic. Season with oregano, red pepper, black pepper, basil and salt.
2. Split the mixture into muffin cups. Lower one cube of cheddar cheese into each meatloaf cup.
3. Close the top to cover the cheese.
4. Bake in the oven at 345°F for 20 minutes, or until the meatloaf cups become golden brown.
5. Let cool for 10 minutes before transferring from the muffin pan.

Nutrition Information:
Calories: 442 kcal— Total Fat: 53g — Total Carbs: 3g— Protein: 26g

6. HAM AND EMMENTAL EGGS

- **1 tbsp olive oil**
- **4 slices ham, chopped**
- **½ cup chives, chopped**
- **½ cup broccoli, chopped**
- **1 clove garlic, minced**
- **1 tsp fines herbes**
- **¼ cup vegetable broth**
- **5 eggs**
- **1 ½ cups Emmental**

cheese, shredded

**TOTAL TIME
20 MINUTES**

DIRECTIONS

1. In a frying pan, warm oil. Add in ham and cook for 4 minutes, until brown and crispy; set aside.
2. Using the same pan, cook chives in pan drippings. Place in the garlic and broccoli and cook until soft as you stir occasionally. Stir in broth and fines herbes and cook for 6 more minutes.
3. Make 5 holes in the vegetable mixture until you are able to see the bottom of your pan.

Crack an egg into each hole. Spread shredded cheese over the top and cook for 6 more minutes. Scatter the reserved ham over, to serve.

Nutrition Information:
Calories: 374 kcal— Total Fat: 20.5g — Total Carbs: 14g— Protein: 26.6g

7. CHEESE, HAM AND EGG MUFFINS

- **24 slices smoked ham**
- **6 eggs, beaten**
- **Salt and black pepper, to taste**
- **¼ cup fresh parsley, chopped**
- **¼ cup ricotta cheese**
- **¼ cup Brie, chopped**

**TOTAL TIME
20 MINUTES**

DIRECTIONS

1. Set oven to 390°F. Line 2 slices of smoked ham to each muffin cup to circle each mold.
2. In a mixing bowl, mix the rest of the ingredients. Fill ¾ of the ham lined muffin cup with the egg/cheese mixture. Bake for 15 minutes. Serve warm!

Nutrition Information:
Calories: 281 kcal— Total Fat: 26g — Total Carbs: 10g— Protein: 17g

8. THREE-CHEESE FONDUE WITH WALNUTS AND PARSLEY

INGREDIENTS

- ½ pound brie cheese, chopped
- ⅓ pound swiss cheese, shredded
- ½ cup emmental cheese, grated
- 1 tbsp xanthan gum
- ½ tsp garlic powder
- 1 tsp onion powder
- ¾ cup white wine
- ½ tbsp lemon juice
- Black pepper, to taste
- 1 cup walnuts, chopped

TOTAL TIME
15 MINUTES

DIRECTIONS

1. Set broiler to preheat. In a skillet, thoroughly mix onion powder, brie, emmental,
2. Swiss cheese, garlic powder, and xanthan gum.
3. Pour in lemon juice and wine and sprinkle with black pepper.
4. Set the skillet under the broiler for 6 to 7 minutes, until the cheese browns. Garnish with walnuts.

Nutrition Information:
Calories: 288 kcal— Total Fat: 18.5g — Total Carbs: 3.5g— Protein: 22g

9. CHEESY BITES WITH TURNIP CHIPS

- **1 cup Monterey Jack cheese, shredded**
- **½ cup natural yogurt**
- **1 cup pecorino cheese, grated**
- **2 tbsp tomato puree**
- **½ tsp dried rosemary leaves, crushed**
- **1 tsp dried thyme leaves, crushed**
- **Salt and black pepper, to taste**
- **1 pound turnips, sliced**
- **2 tbsp olive oil**
- **Salt and black pepper, to taste**

TOTAL TIME
25 MINUTES

DIRECTIONS

1. In a mixing bowl, mix cheese, tomato puree, black pepper, salt, rosemary, yogurt, and thyme. Place in foil liners-candy cups and refrigerate until ready to serve.
2. Set oven to 430°F. Coat turnips with salt, pepper and oil.
3. Arrange in a single layer on a cookie sheet.
4. Bake for 20 minutes, shaking once or twice. Dip turnip chips in cheese cups.

Nutrition Information:
Calories: 495 kcal— Total Fat: 35g — Total Carbs: 6g— Protein: 38g

10. BAKED CHICKEN LEGS WITH CHEESY SPREAD

INGREDIENTS

- **4 chicken legs**
- **¼ cup goat cheese**
- **2 tbsp sour cream**
- **1 tbsp butter, softened**
- **1 onion, chopped**
- **Sea salt and black pepper, to taste**

TOTAL TIME
45 MINUTES

DIRECTIONS

1. Set oven to 360°F.
2. Bake legs for 25-30 minutes until crispy and browned. In a mixing bowl, mix the rest of the ingredients to form the spread.
3. Serve alongside the prepared chicken legs.

Nutrition Information:
Calories: 189 kcal— Total Fat: 18.6g — Total Carbs: 7.5g— Protein: 19.4g

11. JUICY BEEF CHEESEBURGERS

INGREDIENTS

- **1 pound ground beef**
- **½ cup green onions, chopped**
- **2 garlic cloves, finely chopped**
- **¼ tsp black pepper**
- **Sea salt and cayenne pepper, to taste**
- **2 oz mascarpone cheese**
- **3 oz pecorino romano cheese, grated**
- **2 tbsp olive oil**

**TOTAL TIME
20 MINUTES**

DIRECTIONS

1. Using a mixing bowl, mix ground meat, garlic, cayenne pepper, black pepper, green onions, and salt.
2. Shape into 6 balls; then flatten to make burgers.
3. In a separate bowl, mix mascarpone with grated pecorino romano cheese.
4. Split the cheese mixture among prepared patties.
5. Wrap the meat mixture around the cheese to ensure that the filling is sealed inside.
6. Warm oil in a skillet over medium heat. Cook the burgers for 5 minutes each side.

Nutrition Information:
Calories: 189 kcal— Total Fat: 18.6g — Total Carbs: 7.5g— Protein: 19.4g

12. JAMON & QUESO BALLS

INGREDIENTS

- **1 egg**
- **6 slices jamon serrano, chopped**
- **6 ounces cotija cheese**
- **6 ounces Manchego cheese**
- **Salt and black pepper, to taste**
- **¼ cup almond flour**
- **1 tsp baking powder**
- **1 tsp garlic powder**

**TOTAL TIME
15 MINUTES**

DIRECTIONS

1. Set oven to 420 °F.
2. Whisk the eggs; place in the remaining ingredients and mix well.
3. Split the mixture into 16 balls; set the balls on a baking sheet lined with parchment paper.
4. Bake for 13 minutes or until they turn golden brown and become crispy.

Nutrition Information:
Calories: 73 kcal— Total Fat: 11g — Total Carbs: 4g— Protein: 3g

13. CAJUN CRABMEAT FRITTATA

INGREDIENTS

- **1 tbsp olive oil**
- **1 onion, chopped**
- **4 ounces crabmeat, chopped**
- **1 tsp cajun seasoning**
- **6 large eggs, slightly beaten**
- **½ cup Greek yogurt**

TOTAL TIME
25 MINUTES

DIRECTIONS

1. Set oven to 350°F and set a large skillet over medium heat and warm the oil.
2. Add in onion and sauté until soft; place in crabmeat and cook for 2 more minutes. Season with Cajun seasoning.
3. Evenly distribute the ingredients at the bottom of the skillet.
4. Whisk the eggs with yogurt. Transfer to the skillet.
5. Set the skillet in the oven and bake for about 18 minutes or until eggs are cooked through.
6. Slice into wedges and serve warm.

Nutrition Information:
Calories: 299 kcal— Total Fat: 17.6g — Total Carbs: 0.5g— Protein: 33.5g

14. ZUCCHINI WITH BLUE CHEESE AND WALNUTS

- **1 tbsp butter**
- **6 zucchinis, chopped**
- **2 tsp powdered unflavored gelatin**
- **1 ⅓ cups heavy cream**
- **1 cup sour cream**
- **8 ounces blue cheese**
- **1 tsp Italian seasoning**
- **¼ cup walnut halves**

TOTAL TIME
15 MINUTES

DIRECTIONS

1. Set a pan over medium heat and warm butter; add in zucchini and sauté for 4 minutes as you stir. Place in heavy cream and gelatin and cook to boil.
2. Transfer from heat; add the Italian seasoning, cheese and sour cream.
3. Evenly layer the mixture in 6 glasses.
4. Place in the refrigerator for at least 5 hours.
5. Serve decorated with walnut halves.

Nutrition Information:
Calories: 159 kcal— Total Fat: 17.6g — Total Carbs: 8.5g— Protein: 18.5g

15. CHEESE ROLL-UPS THE KETO WAY

INGREDIENTS

- **4 slices cheddar cheese**
- **4 ham slices**

TOTAL TIME
5 MINUTES

DIRECTIONS

1. Place one cheese slice on a flat surface and top with one slice of ham.
2. Roll from one end to the other. Repeat process to remaining cheese and ham.
3. Evenly divide into suggested servings and place in meal prep containers.

Nutrition Information:
Calories: 303 kcal— Total Fat: 28.9g — Total Carbs: 4.6g— Protein: 43.3g

16. SPICED DEVILLED EGGS

- **6 eggs**
- **¼ tsp salt**
- **½ cup mayonnaise**
- **½ tbsp poppy seeds**
- **1 tbsp red curry paste**

TOTAL TIME
13 MINUTES

DIRECTIONS

1. Place eggs in a small pot and add enough water to cover it. Bring to a boil without a cover, lower heat to a simmer and simmer for 8 minutes.
2. Immediately dunk in ice cold water once done cooking. Peel egg shells and slice eggs in half lengthwise.
3. Remove yolks and place them in a medium bowl. Add the rest of the ingredients in the bowl except for the egg whites. Mix well.
4. Evenly return the yolk mixture into the middle of the egg whites.
5. Let it cool. Evenly divide into suggested servings and place in meal prep containers.

Nutrition Information:
Calories: 303 kcal— Total Fat: 28.9g — Total Carbs: 6g— Protein: 33.3g

17. KETO REESE CUPS

INGREDIENTS

- ½ cup unsweetened shredded coconut
- 1 cup almond butter
- 1 cup dark chocolate chips
- 1 tablespoon coconut oil
- 1 tablespoon Stevia

TOTAL TIME
6 MINUTES

DIRECTIONS

1. Line 12 muffin tins with 12 muffin liners.
2. Place the almond butter, honey and oil in a glass bowl and microwave for 30 seconds or until melted. Divide the mixture into 12 muffin tins. Let it cool for 30 minutes in the fridge.
3. Add the shredded coconuts and mix until evenly distributed.
4. Pour the remaining melted chocolate on top of the coconuts. Freeze for an hour.
5. Carefully remove the chocolates from the muffin tins to create perfect Reese cups.
6. Store in airtight meal prep containers.

Nutrition Information:
Calories: 136 kcal— Total Fat: 7g — Total Carbs: 4g— Protein: 19.9g

18. ONION CHEESE MUFFINS

- ¼ cup Colby jack cheese, shredded
- ¼ cup shallots, minced
- ½ tsp salt
- 1 cup almond flour
- 1 egg
- 3 tbsp melted butter
- 3 tbsp sour cream

TOTAL TIME
30 MINUTES

DIRECTIONS

1. Line 6 muffin tins with 6 muffin liners. Set aside and preheat oven to 350oF.
2. In a bowl, stir the dry and wet ingredients alternately. Mix well using a spatula until the consistency of the mixture becomes even.
3. Scoop a spoonful of the batter to the prepared muffin tins.
4. Bake for 20 minutes in oven until golden brown.
5. Let it cool and store in an airtight container.

Nutrition Information:
Calories 387 kcal — Protein 11g — Carbs 9g — Fiber 5g — Fat: 35g

19. BACON-FLAVORED KALE CHIPS

INGREDIENTS

- **1-lb kale, around 1 bunch**
- **1 to 2 tsp salt**
- **2 tbsp butter**
- **¼ cup bacon grease**

TOTAL TIME
35 MINUTES

DIRECTIONS

1. Remove the rib from kale leaves and tear into 2-inch pieces.
2. Clean the kale leaves thoroughly and dry them inside a salad spinner.
3. In a skillet, add the butter to the bacon grease and warm the two fats under low heat. Add salt and stir constantly.
4. Set aside and let it cool.
5. Put the dried kale in a Ziploc back and add the cool liquid bacon grease and butter mixture.
6. Seal the Ziploc back and gently shake the kale leaves with the butter mixture. The leaves should have this shiny consistency which means that they are coated evenly with the fat.
7. Pour the kale leaves on a cookie sheet and sprinkle more salt if necessary.
8. Bake for 25 minutes inside a preheated 350-degree oven or until the leaves start to turn brown as well as crispy.
9. Let it cool, evenly divide into suggested servings and store in an airtight container.

Nutrition Information:
Calories 256g — Total Fat 49g — Total Carbs 8g — Protein: 19g

20. CAULIFLOWER, CHEDDAR & JALAPENO MUFFINS

INGREDIENTS

- **1 cup grated cheddar cheese**
- **1 cup grated mozzarella cheese**
- **1 Tbsp dried onion flakes**
- **1/2 tsp baking powder**
- **1/2 tsp garlic powder**
- **1/3 cup grated parmesan cheese**
- **1/4 cup coconut flour**
- **1/4 tsp black pepper**
- **1/4 tsp salt**
- **2 cups finely riced, raw cauliflower**
- **2 eggs, beaten**
- **2 Tbsp melted butter**
- **2 Tbsp minced jalapeno**

TOTAL TIME
40 MINUTES

DIRECTIONS

1. Line 12 muffin tins with muffin cups and preheat oven to 375oF.
2. In a medium bowl, whisk well eggs. Stir in coconut flour, baking powder, garlic powder, pepper, salt, onion flakes, cheese, melted butter, jalapeno, and cauliflower. Mix thoroughly.
3. Evenly divide into prepared muffin tins.
4. Pop in the oven and bake for 30 minutes.
5. Let it cool. Evenly divide into suggested servings and place in meal prep containers.

Nutrition Information:
Carbs: 7.5g — Calories: 439 — Total Fat: 52.2g — Protein: 12.7g

21. KETO CHOCO-CHIA PUDDING

INGREDIENTS

- **1 tsp Stevia (optional)**
- **¼ cup fresh or frozen raspberries**
- **1 scoop chocolate protein powder**
- **1 cup unsweetened almond milk**
- **3 tbsp Chia seeds**

TOTAL TIME
10 MINUTES

DIRECTIONS

1. Mix the chocolate protein powder and almond milk.
2. Add the chia seeds and mix well with a whisk or a fork.
3. Flavor with Stevia depending on the desired sweetness.
4. Let it rest for 5 minutes and continue stirring.
5. Place in meal prep containers and let it cool in the fridge for at least an hour.

Nutrition Information:
Calories: 112 — Total Fat: 32g — Total Carbs: 5.0g — Protein: 14.3g

22. WALNUT & PUMPKIN SPICE KETO BREAD

INGREDIENTS

- 4 large eggs
- 2 cups almond flour
- 1 tbsp baking powder
- 1 pinch sea salt
- 1 cup pumpkin puree
- 1/2 cup coconut flour (sifted)
- 1/2 cup erythritol
- 1/3 cup heavy cream
- 1/4 cup chopped

- walnuts
- 3/4 cup melted butter
- 1 1/2 tsp pumpkin pie spice

TOTAL TIME
70 MINUTES

DIRECTIONS

1. Lightly grease a loaf pan and preheat oven to 350OF.
2. In a large mixing bowl, whisk well salt, pumpkin spice, baking powder, sugar free sweetener, coconut flour, and almond flour.
3. In a blender, blend until smooth the eggs, heavy cream, butter, and pumpkin.
4. Pour into bowl of dry ingredients and mix thoroughly.

5. Pour batter in loaf pan and bake for 60 minutes or when poked with a toothpick, it comes out clean.
6. Remove bread from pan.
7. Let it cool. Evenly divide into suggested servings and place in meal prep containers.

Nutrition Information:
Calories: 224 kcal — Total Fat: 22g — Total Carbs: 8.2g — Protein: 23.5 g

23. LOW CARB KETO PEANUT BUTTER COOKIES

INGREDIENTS

- 2 large eggs
- ¼ tsp salt
- 1 cup unsweetened peanut butter
- 1 tsp baking soda
- 1 tsp stevia powder
- 1/8 tsp xanthan gum
- 2 cups almond flour
- 2 tbsp butter
- 2 tsp pure vanilla
- extract
- 4 ounces softened cream cheese
- 5 drops liquid Splenda

TOTAL TIME
20 MINUTES

DIRECTIONS

1. Line a cookie sheet with a non-stick liner. Set aside.
2. In a bowl, mix xanthan gum, flour, salt and baking soda. Set aside.
3. On a mixing bowl, combine the butter, cream cheese and peanut butter.
4. Mix on high speed until it forms a smooth consistency. Add the sweetener. Add the eggs and vanilla gradually while mixing until it forms a smooth consistency.
5. Add the almond flour mixture slowly and mix until well combined.
6. The dough is ready once it starts to stick together into a ball.
7. Scoop the dough using a 1 tablespoon cookie scoop and drop each cookie on the prepared cookie sheet. You will make around 24 cookies
8. Press the cookie with a fork and bake for 10 to 12 minutes at 350OF.
9. Let it cool and place in an airtight container.

Nutrition Information:
Calories 231 kcal — Protein: 26.7g — Carbs: 4.8g — Fat 74g

24. NO COOK COCONUT AND CHOCOLATE BARS

INGREDIENTS

- **1 tbsp Stevia**
- **¾ cup shredded coconut, unsweetened**
- **½ cup ground nuts (almonds, pecans, or walnuts)**
- **¼ cup unsweetened cocoa powder**
- **4 tbsps coconut oil**

TOTAL TIME
6 MINUTES

DIRECTIONS

1. In a medium bowl, mix shredded coconut, nuts and cocoa powder.
2. Add Stevia and coconut oil.
3. Mix batter thoroughly.
4. In a 9x9 square inch pan or dish, press the batter and for 30-minutes place in the freezer.
5. Evenly divide into suggested servings and place in meal prep containers.

Nutrition Information:
Calories: 364 Kcal — Total Carbs: 2.5g — Total Fat: 55.5g — Protein: 13.5g

25. KETO-APPROVED TRAIL MIX

INGREDIENTS

- **½ cup salted pumpkin seeds**
- **½ cup slivered almonds**
- **¾ cup roasted pecan halves**
- **¾ cup unsweetened cranberries**
- **1 cup toasted coconut flakes**

TOTAL TIME
8 MINUTES

DIRECTIONS

1. In a skillet, place almonds and pecans. Heat for 2-3 minutes and let cool.
2. Once cooled, in a large re-sealable plastic bag, combine all ingredients.
3. Seal and shake vigorously to mix.
4. Evenly divide into suggested servings and store in airtight meal prep containers.

Nutrition Information:
Calories: 224 kcal — Total Fat: 22g — Total Carbs: 8.2g — Protein: 23.5 g

26. BACON AND CHEDDAR CHEESE BALLS

- **5 1/3-oz bacon**
- **5 1/3-oz cheddar cheese**
- **5 1/3-oz cream cheese**
- **½ tsp chili flakes (optional)**
- **½ tsp pepper (optional)**

TOTAL TIME
15 MINUTES

DIRECTIONS

1. Pan fry bacon until crisped, around 8 minutes.
2. Meanwhile, in a food processor, process remaining ingredients. Then transfer to a bowl and refrigerate. When ready to handle, form into 20 equal balls.
3. Once bacon is cooked, crumble bacon and spread on a plate.
4. Roll the balls on the crumbled bacon to coat.
5. Store in airtight meal prep containers.

Nutrition Information:
Calories: 287 kcal — Total Fat: 19g — Total Carbs: 6.5g — Protein: 6.8g

27. FLAXSEED, MAPLE & PUMPKIN MUFFIN

INGREDIENTS

- 1 tbsp cinnamon
- 1 cup pure pumpkin puree
- 1 tbsp pumpkin pie spice
- 2 tbsp coconut oil
- 1 egg
- 1/2 tbsp baking powder
- 1/2 tsp salt
- 1/2 tsp apple cider vinegar
- 1/2 tsp vanilla extract
- 1/3 cup erythritol
- 1 1/4 cup flaxseeds (ground)
- 1/4 cup Walden Farm's Maple Syrup

TOTAL TIME
30 MINUTES

DIRECTIONS

1. Line ten muffin tins with ten muffin liners and preheat oven to 350oF.
2. In a blender, add all ingredients and blend until smooth and creamy, around 5 minutes.
3. Evenly divide batter into prepared muffin tins.
4. Pop in the oven and bake for 20 minutes or until tops are lightly browned.
5. Let it cool. Evenly divide into suggested servings and place in meal prep containers.

Nutrition Information:
Calories: 202.5kal; protein 15.8g; Carbohydrate: 20.6g; Fat 7g.

28. GARLICK & CHEESE TURKEY SLICES

- **1 tbsp olive oil**
- **1 pound turkey breasts, sliced**
- **2 garlic cloves, minced**
- **½ cup heavy cream**
- **⅓ cup chicken broth**
- **2 tbsp tomato paste**
- **1 cup cheddar cheese, shredded**

**TOTAL TIME
20 MINUTES**

DIRECTIONS

1. Set a pan over medium heat and warm the oil; add in garlic and turkey and fry for 4 minutes; set aside.
2. Stir in the broth, tomato paste, and heavy cream; cook until thickened.
3. Return the turkey to the pan; spread shredded cheese over. Let sit for 5 minutes while covered or until the cheese melts.
4. Place in the refrigerator for a maximum of 3 days or serve instantly.
Nutrition Information:
Calories: 97.2kal; protein 7.8g; Carbohydrate: 16.2g; Fat 7g

29. PROSCIUTTO & CHEESE EGG CUPS

- **9 slices prosciutto**
- **9 eggs**
- **4 green onions, chopped**
- **½ cup cheddar cheese, shredded**
- **¼ tsp garlic powder**
- **½ tsp dried dill weed**
- **Sea salt and black pepper, to taste**

**TOTAL TIME
30 MINUTES**

DIRECTIONS

1. Set oven to 390°F and grease a 9-cup muffin pan with oil.
2. Line one slice of prosciutto on each cup.
3. In a mixing bowl, combine the remaining ingredients.
4. Split the egg mixture among muffin cups.
5. Bake for 20 minutes. Leave to cool before serving.

Nutrition Information:
Calories: 120 kal; protein 13.4g; Carbohydrate: 14.4g; Fat 7g.

30. CILANTRO & CHILI OMELET

- **2 tsp butter**
- **2 spring onions, chopped**
- **2 spring garlic, chopped**
- **4 eggs, beaten**
- **1 cup sour cream, divided**
- **2 tomatoes, sliced**
- **1 green chili pepper,**
- **minced**
- **2 tbsp fresh cilantro, chopped**
- **Salt and black pepper, to taste**

TOTAL TIME
15 MINUTES

DIRECTIONS

1. Set a pan over high heat and warm the butter. Sauté garlic and onions until tender and translucent.
2. Whisk the eggs with sour cream. Pour into the pan and use a spatula to smooth the surface; cook until eggs become puffy and brown to bottom.
3. Add cilantro, chili pepper and tomatoes to one side of the omelet.
4. Add in pepper and salt. Fold the omelet in half and slice into wedges.

Nutrition Information:
328 calories; 14.8 g total fat; 37.5 g carbohydrates; 2.7 g fiber; 14.1 g protein;

31. BACON BALLS WITH BRIE CHEESE

- **3 ounces bacon**
- **6 ounces goat's cheese**
- **1 chili pepper, seeded and chopped**
- **¼ tsp parsley flakes**
- **½ tsp paprika**

TOTAL TIME
15 MINUTES

DIRECTIONS

1. Set a frying pan over medium heat and fry the bacon until crispy; then chop it into small pieces.
2. Place the other ingredients in a bowl and mix to combine well. Refrigerate the mixture.
3. Create balls from the mixture.
4. Set the crushed bacon in a plate.
5. Roll the balls around to coat all sides.

Nutrition Information:
Calories: 210g; Fat: 10g; carbohydrates: 27g; 2.7 g fiber: 4g; sugar; 1.6g protein: 3.7g

32. CREAMY CHEDDAR DEVILED EGGS

INGREDIENTS

- **10 eggs**
- **¼ cup mayonnaise**
- **1 tbsp tomato paste**
- **2 tbsp celery, chopped**
- **2 tbsp carrot, chopped**
- **2 tbsp chives, minced**
- **2 tbsp cheddar cheese, grated**
- **Salt and black pepper, to taste**

TOTAL TIME
20 MINUTES

DIRECTIONS

1. Place the eggs in a pot and fill with water by about 1 inch.
2. Bring the eggs to a boil over high heat, then reduce the heat to medium and simmer for 10 minutes.
3. Remove and rinse under running water until cooled.
4. Peel and discard the shell. Slice each egg in half lengthwise and get rid of the yolks.
5. Mix the yolks with the rest of the ingredients.
6. Split the mixture amongst the egg whites and set deviled eggs on a plate to serve.

Nutrition Information:
Calories: 270g; Fat: 9g; carbohydrates: 40g; 2.7 g; sugar; 24g protein: 20.5g

33. GINGERY TUNA MOUSSE

- 1 ½ tsp gelatin, powdered
- 3 tbsp water
- 2 ounces ricotta cheese
- 3 tbsp mayonnaise
- 1 tsp mustard
- 3 ounces canned tuna, flaked
- ¼ cup onions, chopped
- 1 garlic clove, minced
- ½ tsp salt
- ¼ tsp black pepper
- ⅓ tsp ginger, grated

TOTAL TIME
20 MINUTES

DIRECTIONS

1. Mix gelatin in water; let sit for 10 minutes.
2. Set a pan over medium heat and warm ricotta cheese; place in gelatin and mix to blend well; let the mixture cool.
3. Place in the other ingredients and stir.
4. Split the mixture among 5 mousse molds and refrigerate overnight.
5. Serve by inverting the molds over a serving platter.

Nutrition Information:
Calories: 120g Fat: 10g ; carbohydrates: 15g; protein: 27g;

34. MINI EGG MUFFINS

- **1 tbsp olive oil**
- **1 onion, chopped**
- **1 bell pepper, chopped**
- **6 slices bacon, chopped**
- **8 eggs, whisked**
- **1 cup gruyere cheese, shredded**
- **Salt and black pepper, to taste**
- **¼ tsp rosemary**
- **1 tbsp fresh parsley, chopped**

TOTAL TIME
40 MINUTES

DIRECTIONS

1. Set oven to 390°F. Place cupcake liners to your muffin pan.
2. In a skillet over medium heat, warm the oil and sauté the onions and bell pepper for 4-5 minutes, as you stir constantly until tender.
3. Stir in bacon and cook for 3 more minutes.
4. Add in the rest of the ingredients and mix well.
5. Set the mixture to the lined muffin pan and bake for 23 minutes; let muffins cool, before serving.

Nutrition Information:
Calories: 147 — Total Fat: 21g — Total Carbs: 3.5g — Protein: 6.8g

35. GRILLED HALLOUMI CHEESE WITH EGGS

INGREDIENTS

- **4 slices halloumi cheese**
- **3 tsp olive oil**
- **1 tsp dried Greek seasoning blend**
- **1 tbsp olive oil**
- **6 eggs, beaten**
- **½ tsp sea salt**
- **¼ tsp crushed red pepper flakes**
- **1 ½ cups avocado, pitted and sliced**
- **1 cup grape tomatoes, halved**
- **4 tbsp pecans, chopped**

TOTAL TIME
20 MINUTES

DIRECTIONS

1. Preheat your grill to medium.
2. Set the Halloumi in the center of a piece of heavy-duty foil.
3. Sprinkle oil over the Halloumi and apply Greek seasoning blend.
4. Close the foil to create a packet.
5. Grill for about 15 minutes; then slice into four pieces.
6. In a frying pan, warm 1 tablespoon of oil and cook the eggs.
7. Stir well to create large and soft curds. Season with salt and pepper.
8. Put the eggs and grilled cheese on a serving bowl.
9. Serve alongside tomatoes and avocado, decorated with chopped pecans.

Nutrition Information:
Calories: 700 kcal — Total Fat: 40g — Total Carbs: 4g — Protein: 30g

36. CHORIZO AND CHEESE GOFRE

INGREDIENTS

- **6 eggs, separate egg whites and egg yolks**
- **½ tsp baking powder**
- **½ tsp baking soda**
- **4 tbsp butter**
- **Salt to taste**
- **½ tsp dried rosemary**
- **3 tbsp tomato puree**
- **3 ounces smoked chorizo, chopped**

- **3 ounces cheddar cheese, shredded**

TOTAL TIME
20 MINUTES

DIRECTIONS

1. In a mixing bowl, mix egg yolks, baking soda, oregano, ghee, baking powder, and salt. Beat the egg whites until pale and combine with the egg yolk mixture.
2. Grease waffle iron and set over medium heat, add in ¼ cup of the batter and cook for 3 minutes until golden. Do the same with the remaining batter until you have 6 thin waffles.
3. Place one waffle back to the waffle iron; sprinkle 1 tablespoon of tomato puree to the waffle; apply a topping of 1 ounce of shredded cheese and 1 ounce of chorizo.
4. Cover with another waffle; cook until all the cheese melts. Do the same with all remaining ingredients.

Nutrition Information:
Calories: 103 kcal — Total Fat: 30g — Total Carbs: 4.8g — Protein: 13.9g

37. CRÊPES WITH LEMON-BUTTERY SYRUP

- **For Crêpes:**
- **6 ounces mascarpone cheese, softened**
- **6 eggs**
- **1 ½ tbsp granulated swerve**
- **¼ cup almond flour**
- **1 tsp baking soda**
- **1 tsp baking powder**
- **For the Syrup**

- **¾ cup water**
- **2 tbsp lemon juice**
- **1 tbsp butter**
- **¾ cup swerve, powdered**
- **1 tbsp vanilla extract**
- **½ tsp xanthan gum**

TOTAL TIME
25 MINUTES

DIRECTIONS

1. With the use of an electric mixer, mix all crepes ingredients until well incorporated.
2. Use melted butter to grease a frying pan and set over medium heat; cook the crepes until the edges start to brown, about 2 minutes. Flip over and cook the other side for a further 2 minutes; repeat the process with the remaining batter. Put the crepes on a plate.

3. In the same pan, mix swerve, butter and water; simmer for 6 minutes as you stir. Transfer the mixture to a blender together with a ¼ teaspoon of xanthan gum and vanilla extract and mix well. Place in the remaining ¼ teaspoon of xanthan gum and allow to sit until the syrup is thick.

Nutrition Information:
Calories: 632 kcal — Total Fat: 43g — Total Carbs: 15g — Protein: 49g

38. CHILI EGG PICKLES

- **10 eggs**
- **½ cup onions, sliced**
- **3 cardamom pods**
- **1 tbsp chili powder**
- **1 tsp yellow seeds**
- **2 clove garlic, sliced**
- **1 cup vinegar**
- **1 ¼ cups water**
- **1 tbsp salt**

TOTAL TIME
20 MINUTES

DIRECTIONS

1. Boil eggs in salted water until hard-cooked, about 10 minutes; rinse under cold, running water; peel and discard the shell.
2. Place the peeled eggs onto a large jar.
3. Set a pan over medium heat. Stir in all remaining ingredients; bring to a rapid boil.
4. Reduce heat to low; allow to simmer for 6 minutes. Spoon this mixture into the jar.
5. Refrigerate for 2 to 3 weeks.

Nutrition Information:
Calories: 448 kcal — Total Fat: 40.3g — Total Carbs: 2.8g — Protein: 16.9g

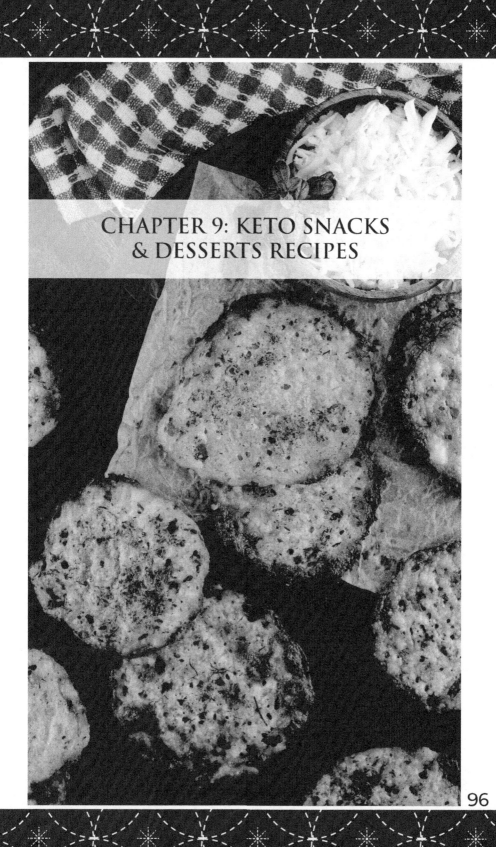

CHAPTER 9: KETO SNACKS
& DESSERTS RECIPES

1. KETO CHOCO-VANILLA MUFFINS

- **1 cup almond flour**
- **1/2 cup erythritol**
- **1/2 cup cocoa powder**
- **1 1/2 tsp baking powder**
- **1 tsp vanilla extract**
- **3 eggs**
- **2/3 cup heavy cream**
- **3 oz butter**
- **1/2 cup sugar free chocolate chips**

TOTAL TIME
30 MINUTES

DIRECTIONS

1. In a bowl add almond flour, cocoa powder, erythritol and baking powder.
2. Pour vanilla extract, eggs and cream and mix well until combined.
3. Now add butter and chocolate chips and stir well. Take muffin baking tray and pour the mixture into it.
4. Bake it for 20 minutes on preheated oven at 175C until puffed.
5. Let them cool and serve.

Nutrition Information:
Calories: 391.25 kcal— Total Fat: 15.5g — Total Carbs: 43.4g— Protein: 11.4g

2. HOMEMADE THIN MINTS (LOW CARB AND GLUTEN FREE)

- **For cookies:**
- **¼ cup natural sweetener**
- **1 teaspoon baking powder**
- **1 ¾ cups almond flour**
- **1/3 cup cocoa powder**
- **¼ teaspoon salt**
- **1 large egg beaten**
- **1/8 teaspoon liquid stevia**
- **2 tablespoon butter**

- **½ teaspoon vanilla extract**
-
- **For Coating:**
- **1 teaspoon peppermint extract**
- **200 gram dark chocolate**
- **1 tablespoon butter**

TOTAL TIME
60 MINUTES

DIRECTIONS

1. Cookies:
2. Preheat the oven to 180°C.
3. And line baking tray with parchment baking paper. In a bowl, mix cocoa powder, almond flour, natural sweetener, baking powder and salt.
4. Also add stevia liquid, egg, butter and vanilla extract and mix well until dough is combined.
5. Now make Cookies of 2 inch diameter. P
6. lace cookies on prepared baking tray. Bake cookies

for almost 15 to 20 minutes.
7. Remove and let cool.
8. Coating:
9. Take a pan melt the coconut oil and chocolate, mix until smooth.
10. Remove from flame and add in the peppermint extract.
11. Let the mixture cool.
12. Dip the cookies into the mixture; make sure both sides are coated well.
13. Refrigerate until fully set.

Nutrition Information:
Calories: 241 kcal— Total Fat: 22.1g — Total Carbs: 1.5g— Protein: 10.1g

3. DARK CHOCOLATE COVERED WALNUTS

INGREDIENTS

- **2 cups shelled walnuts**
- **1/2 cup unsweetened chocolate chopped**
- **¼ cup powdered Stevia or any other natural sweetener**
- **3 tablespoon walnut oil**
- **½ teaspoon vanilla extract**
- **1 tablespoon**

unsweetened cocoa powder

TOTAL TIME
30 MINUTES

DIRECTIONS

1. Take a pan; combine chocolate, powdered.
2. Swerve, and walnut oil on low heat.
3. Stir well until melted and smooth.
4. Now add in vanilla extract and cocoa powder until smooth.
5. Let the mixture cool for 5 minutes to thicken.
6. Now dip walnuts in the chocolate mixture, do the same with all walnuts.
7. Place walnuts on baking sheet and chill in freezer until firm.
8. They Can be stored an airtight container for few days.

Nutrition Information:
Cholesterol: 326mg— Total Fat: 16g — Total Carbs: 4g— Protein: 11.5g4g

4. CHOCOLATE COCONUT KETO SMOOTHIE BOWL

INGREDIENTS

- 1/3 cup vanilla protein powder
- 1/2 cup almond milk
- 1 tbsp cocoa powder
- 1 tbsp coconut oil
- Sweetener
- 3 cup crushed ice
- 1/8 tsp xanthan gum
- 1/2 cup raspberries
- 1/4 cup walnuts
- 2 tbsp pomegranate

TOTAL TIME
10 MINUTES

DIRECTIONS

1. Take a blender pour almond milk, protein powder, cocoa powder, sweetener and ice, blend the ingredients well.
2. Now add coconut oil xanthan gum and blend until it increases in volume.
3. Pour it into bowl adds fruits and nuts and serves.

Nutrition Information:
Cholesterol: 326mg— Total Fat: 16g — Total Carbs: 4g— Protein: 11.5g4g

5. HOMEMADE GRAHAM CRACKERS

INGREDIENTS

- **1½ cups almond flour**
- **1⅓cups graham flour**
- **1 teaspoon baking soda**
- **½ teaspoon salt**
- **2 Tablespoon unsalted butter**
- **2/3 cups dark brown sugar**
- **Vanilla extract**
- **1 egg**

TOTAL TIME
60 MINUTES

DIRECTIONS

1. Preheat oven to 180°C. In a bowl, beat graham flour, almond flour, sweetener, baking powder and salt.
2. Blend in vanilla extract, egg and melted butter until dough becomes a mixture.
3. Make rough rectangles of the dough.
4. Use knife or a pizza wheel to cut into squares of about 2x2 inches.
5. Transfer the pieces to a baking sheet. Bake 20 to 30 minutes, until golden brown.
6. Take them out and let them cool again.
7. Enjoy crispy crackers.

Nutrition Information:
Carbs: 8; Calories: 200; Total Fat: 9g; Protein: 25g;

6. BLACKENED TILAPIA WITH ZUCCHINI NOODLES

INGREDIENTS

- 2 zucchini, sliced
- ¾ teaspoon salt
- 2 garlic cloves, chomped
- 1 cup Pico de Gallo
- 1 ½ pounds fish
- 2 teaspoons olive oil
- ½ teaspoon cumin, crushed
- ¼ teaspoon garlic powder
- ½ paprika, smoked
- ½ teaspoon pepper

TOTAL TIME
35 MINUTES

DIRECTIONS

1. In a bowl add half salt, pepper, cumin, paprika, and garlic powder, mix them well and sprinkle it on each side of the fish thoroughly.
2. Heat the oil over the medium-heat flame in a nonstick pan.
3. Cook the fish for 3 minutes per side and remove from the pan.
4. Cook zucchini and garlic, remaining salt in the same pan over the medium-high flame for 2 minutes and stir continuously and it's ready to serve.

Nutrition Information:
Carbs: 8; Calories: 200; Total Fat: 10g; Protein: 22.1g; Sugar: 0g; Fibers: 2.1g

7. BELL PEPPER NACHOS

- **2 bell peppers, without stem and seeds**
- **4 ounces beef ground**
- **¼ teaspoon cumin, crushed**
- **¼ cup guacamole**
- **A pinch of salt**
- **1 cup cheese**
- **¼ teaspoon chili powder**
- **1 tablespoon vegetable oil**
- **2 tablespoons sour cream**
- **¼ cup Pico de Gallo**

TOTAL TIME
35 MINUTES

DIRECTIONS

1. Place the bell peppers without stem and seeds in a microwave dish, sprinkle salt and splash water on it and microwave it for 4 minutes and cut it in 4 pieces from sides.
2. Heat oil in a medium flame in a nonstick pan. Toast the chili powder and cumin in this for 30 seconds.
3. Put the beef with salt in it, stir and cook it for 4 minutes. Put this mixture on all the pieces of pepper.
4. Add cheese on it and cook it for 1 minute to melt the cheese.
5. On its top add Pico de Gallo, guacamole, and cream on it.

Nutrition Information:
Calories: 160 kals; Fat: 1 gram; Carbohydrates: 13 grams; Dietary Fiber: 2 grams; Protein: 25 grams.

8. RADISH, CARROT & CILANTRO SALAD

INGREDIENTS

- **1 ½ pounds carrots, sliced**
- **¼ cup cilantro**
- **1 ½ pound radish, sliced**
- **½ teaspoon salt**
- **6 onions, minced**
- **¼ teaspoon black pepper**
- **3 tablespoons lemon juice**
- **3 tablespoons orange juice**
- **2 tablespoons olive oil**

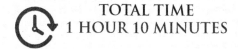

TOTAL TIME
1 HOUR 10 MINUTES

DIRECTIONS

1. Take a big bowl and add all the ingredients in it toast and mix all the ingredients until they merged properly.
2. Put this bowl in the refrigerator for at least one hour to chill and then it is ready to serve.

Nutrition Information:
Calories grams: 240 kals; Carbohydrate: 25 grams, Protein: 26 grams;
Fat: 3.5; Fibre: 4 grams;

9. ASPARAGUS-MUSHROOM FRITTATA

- **1 tablespoon olive oil**
- **1garlic clove, chopped**
- **¼ cup onion, sliced**
- **2 cups white button mushrooms, sliced**
- **1 bunch asparagus**
- **1 tablespoon thyme**
- **6 eggs**
- **½ cup feta cheese, diced**
- **A pinch of salt and black pepper**

TOTAL TIME
35 MINUTES

DIRECTIONS

1. In a pan heat the olive oil over the medium flame, add onions in it and cook for 5 minutes.
2. In this add mushroom and garlic and cook for 5 minutes more.
3. Mix thyme, salt, pepper, and asparagus in it and cook for an additional 3 minutes.
4. Beat eggs and cheese in a bowl and pour it in the pan and cook for 2 to 3 minutes.
5. And finally, transfer it in the greased dish and put it in the 400 degrees F preheated oven to bake for around 10 minutes.

Nutrition Information:
Calories: 445 kcal— Total Fat: 32g — Total Carbs: 9g— Protein: 21g

10. SHRIMP AVOCADO SALAD

- 1/4 cup chopped onion
- 1 medium tomato
- 2 limes juice
- 1medium avocado
- 1/4 tsp salt and black pepper
- 1 jalapeno without seeds
- 1lb peeled shrimp cooked

- 1 tbsp chopped cilantro

TOTAL TIME
20 MINUTES

DIRECTIONS

1. Take a bowl and add onion, lime juice, salt and pepper and mix well or leave it for at least 5 minutes.
2. Now in another bowl add shopped shrimp, avocado, tomato and jalapeno and add onion mixture into them.
3. Combine well and add salt and pepper as per taste, toss and serve.

Nutrition Information:
Calories: 546 kcal— Total Fat: 32g — Total Carbs: 50g— Protein: 32g

11. SMOKY CAULIFLOWER BITES

- **1 large cauliflower**
- **2 garlic cloves**
- **2tbsp olive oil**
- **2 tbsp minced fresh parsley**
- **1tsp paprika**
- **3/4 tsp salt**

TOTAL TIME
40 MINUTES

DIRECTIONS

1. Cut the cauliflower and put into a bowl.
2. Add olive oil, paprika and salt and toss well. Preheat oven at 450.
3. Put the cauliflower mixture in baking pan and bake for at least 10 minutes.
4. After that add garlic and again put in oven for 10 to 15 minutes until it turn brown.
5. Now dish out and sprinkle with parsley and serve.

Nutrition Information:
Calories: 158 kcal— Total Fat: 64g — Total Carbs: 5g— Protein: 22g

12. AVOCADO CRAB BOATS

INGREDIENTS

- **12oz lump crab meat**
- **3tbsp lemon juice**
- **1/3 cup Greek yogurt**
- **1/2 tsp pepper**
- **1/2 minced onion**
- **Salt**
- **2tbsp chopped chives**
- **1 cup shredded cheddar cheese**
- **2 avocados**

TOTAL TIME
10 MINUTES

DIRECTIONS

1. Take a bowl and add meat, yogurt, onion, chives, lemon juice, cayenne and salt to taste, mix them well.
2. Take 2 avocados center half and pitted.
3. Scoop out the avocado from inside and create a bowl, fill avocado bowl with meat mixture and top with cheddar cheese.
4. Now put them into preheat boiler for 2 minutes until cheese melt and serve.

Nutrition Information:
Calories: 687 kcal— Total Fat: 59g — Total Carbs: 2g— Protein: 39g

13. COCONUT CURRY CAULIFLOWER SOUP

INGREDIENTS

- 1tbsp olive oil
- 2-3 tsp curry powder
- 1 medium onion
- 2tsp ground cumin
- 3 garlic cloves
- 1/2 tsp turmeric powder
- 1 tsp ginger
- 14 oz coconut milk
- 14 oz tomatoes
- 1 cup vegetable broth
- 1 cauliflower
- Salt and pepper

TOTAL TIME
35 MINUTES

DIRECTIONS

1. Take a pot adds olive oil and onion and set it on medium flam for sauté.
2. After 3 minutes add garlic, ginger, curry powder, cumin and turmeric powder and sauté for more 5 minutes.
3. Now add coconut milk, tomatoes, vegetable broth and cauliflower and mix it well. Let the mixture heat and bring to boil.
4. Now on low flam cook it for at least 20 minutes until cauliflower turn into soft, blend the mixture well through blender and heat the soup for more 5 minutes and add salt and pepper as per taste, serve the hot seasonal soup.

Nutrition Information:
Calories: 452 kcal— Total Fat: 39g — Total Carbs: 5g— Protein: 19.5g

14. PARMESAN ASPARAGUS

- **4lb fresh asparagus**
- **Salt to taste**
- **1/4 lb butter**
- **2 cups parmesan cheese shredded**
- **1/2 tsp pepper**

TOTAL TIME
32 MINUTES

DIRECTIONS

1. Cut the asparagus and boil it into a large saucepan for almost 3 minutes.
2. After that drain the water and set it aside.
3. Preheat oven at 350. Take a baking pan and grease it well.
4. Evenly arrange asparagus into the pan and pour butter, sprinkle pepper, sale and parmesan cheese.
5. Bake it for almost 10 to 15 minutes until cheese melt. Serve and enjoy.

Nutrition Information:
Calories: 245 kcal— Total Fat: 32g — Total Carbs: 15g— Protein: 16g

15. CREAM CHEESE PANCAKES

INGREDIENTS

- **4 oz cream cheese**
- **Vanilla extract or cinnamon**
- **4 eggs**
- **Butter for grease**

TOTAL TIME
15 MINUTES

DIRECTIONS

1. Take an electric blender adds cream cheese and eggs into it and beat well until mixture turn smooth.
2. Set mixture aside for few minutes.
3. Now heat skilled and grease with butter.
4. Take 1/8 cup of mixture and pour it into skilled.
5. Cook for a minute and then flip and cook another side for a minute and dish out in plate.
6. Make 12 to 14 pancakes and serve with sprinkle cinnamon or sugar dust and enjoy.

Nutrition Information:
Calories: 229 kcal— Total Fat: 49g — Total Carbs: 15g— Protein: 26g

16. COCONUT CHIA PUDDING

- **1/4 cup chia seeds**
- **1 1/4 cup coconut milk**
- **2 tbsp unsweetened coconut**
- **1 tsp vanilla extract**
- **2 tbsp maple syrup**

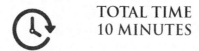

TOTAL TIME
10 MINUTES

DIRECTIONS

1. Soak chia seeds in water for 2 to 3 minutes.
2. Take a bowl add coconut milk, maple syrup, vanilla extract and chia seeds and whisk them well.
3. Let it aside and mix again after 5 minutes.
4. Put it in air tight bar and place in refrigerator for 1 hour.
5. Serve and enjoy chilled coconut chia pudding.

Nutrition Information:
Calories: 243 kcal— Total Fat: 31g — Total Carbs: 4.5g — Protein: 17g

17. SUGAR-FREE MEXICAN SPICED DARK CHOCOLATE

INGREDIENTS

- **1/2 cup cocoa powder**
- **1/4 tsp cinnamon**
- **1/2 tsp chili powder**
- **1/8 tsp nutmeg**
- **1 pinch black pepper**
- **1 pinch salt**
- **1/4 cup melted butter**
- **1/4 tsp vanilla extract**
- **25 drops liquid stevia to taste**

TOTAL TIME
10 MINUTES

DIRECTIONS

1. Take a small bowl mix cocoa powder, cinnamon, chili powder, nutmeg, black pepper and salt together.
2. Set it aside.
3. Stir melted butter with vanilla extract and stevia and mix butter mixture with dry ingredients well until smooth.
4. Put the mixture in chocolate molds and let it set at room temperature until firm.
5. Store in freezer or at room temperature in air tight container.

Nutrition Information:
Calories: 297 kcal— Total Fat: 49g — Total Carbs: 9g— Protein: 30g

18. LOW CARB NO-BAKE CHOCOLATE CHEESECAKE

- 2 oz unsalted butter
- 3.5 oz almond flour
- 3.5 oz sugar free chocolate
- 3.5 oz shredded coconut
- 1 tbsp natvia

Filling
- 7 oz sugar free chocolate
- 8 oz cream cheese
- 3.5 oz natvia
- 1 tsp vanilla extract
- 2 tbsp cocoa powder
- 5.5 oz heavy whipping cream

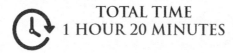

TOTAL TIME
1 HOUR 20 MINUTES

DIRECTIONS

1. For base: take a bowl, add chocolate and butter and set on a pan of boiling water to melt.
2. After that add almond flour, cocon
3. ut and natvia and mix them well.
4. Put the mixture in the cake pan and press it well and freeze until topping prepared.
5. For filling: add chocolate in a bowl and put on a pan with boiling water to melt. In another bowl add cream cheese, natvia, vanilla extract and whipping cream and mix well.
6. Now add cocoa powder and mix until smooth.
7. After that pour melted chocolate and combine all ingredients well.
8. Pour mixture on the base and set it in freezer for an hour.
9. Serve and enjoy chilled keto chocolate cheese cake.

Nutrition Information:
Calories: 360 kcal— Total Fat: 28g — Total Carbs: 3.1g— Protein: 21g

19. KETO HEALTHY MINT CHOCOLATE FUDGE

INGREDIENTS

- **Chocolate layer:**
- 1 1/4 cup heavy cream
- 1/2 cup powdered swerve
- 1/4 tsp liquid stevia
- 1/2 tsp vanilla extract
- 6 oz unsweetened chocolate

- **Mint layer:**
- 8 oz cream cheese
- 1/4 cup powdered swerve
- 2 tbsp heavy cream
- 1 1/2 tsp mint extract
- 1/2 tsp matcha powder

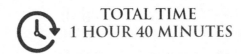

TOTAL TIME
1 HOUR 40 MINUTES

DIRECTIONS

1. Take a pan and add cream and powdered swerve and heat on medium flam until boil.
2. After removing from stove add vanilla extract and stevia and mix, now add chocolate and mix until it melts and turn smooth.
3. Take a pan and place parchment paper in it.
4. Pour chocolate mixture and place in freezer for 20 minutes.
5. Now take a bowl add cream cheese, sweetener, mint extract, heavy cream and matcha powder and whisk well.
6. Pour the mixture on chocolate layer and put in freezer for an hour.

Nutrition Information:
Calories: 360 kcal— Total Fat: 28g — Total Carbs: 3.1g— Protein: 21g

20. ALMOND KETO SHORTBREAD COOKIES

INGREDIENTS

- 1/3 cup coconut flour
- 1/4 cup erythritol
- 2/3 cup almond flour
- 8 drops stevia
- 1/2 cup butter
- 1 tsp almond or vanilla extract
- 1/4 tsp baking powder

- **For glaze:**
- 1/4 cup coconut butter
- 8 drops stevia

TOTAL TIME
21 MINUTES

DIRECTIONS

1. In a bowl add coconut flour, almond flour, erythritol, baking powder and add vanilla or almond extract, stevia and melted butter and make soft dough.
2. Divide dough into two balls and put in refrigerator for 10 minutes. Roll dough on a sheet and cut cookies with help of cookie cutter.
3. Place cookies into a baking pan and bake for 6 minutes in preheated oven at 180C.
4. Now let the cookies completely cool and apply glaze.

Nutrition Information:
Calories: 421 kcal— Total Fat: 42g — Total Carbs: 9g— Protein: 20g

21. MAGIC KETO COOKIES

- **1/4 cup coconut oil**
- **3 tbsp sweetener**
- **4 tbsp unsalted butter**
- **1 cup sugar free chocolate chips**
- **1 cup coconut flakes**
- **1/2 cup pecans**
- **1/2 cup walnuts**
- **1 tsp vanilla extract**
- **4 egg yolks**

- **Sea salt**

TOTAL TIME
22 MINUTES

DIRECTIONS

1. Take a bowl and mix coconut oil, butter, sweetener, chocolate chips, vanilla extract, egg yolks, coconut and walnuts and stir well.
2. Use a scope to make cookie and drop even amount of dough on baking pan.
3. Sprinkle salt as per taste and bake for 12 minutes on preheated oven at 350F until golden brown.

Nutrition Information:
Calories: 300 kcal— Total Fat: 30 — Total Carbs: 10g— Protein: 4g

22. LOW CARB CHOCOLATE PIZZA

INGREDIENTS

- 1 3/4 cup almond flour
- 1/3 cup bocha sweet
- 1/3 cup cocoa powder
- 1 tsp baking powder
- 1/4 tsp salt
- 1 egg
- 2 tbsp butter
- 1/2 vanilla extract

Cream cheese frosting
- 4 oz cream cheese

- 1/4 cup powdered bocha sweet
- 2 tbsp heavy cream
- 1/2 tsp vanilla extract
- Topping
- 5 strawberries
- 1/4 cup blueberries
- 1/4 cup whipping cream
- 1 oz sugar free chocolate chips

TOTAL TIME
60 MINUTES

DIRECTIONS

1. Chocolate crust: take a bowl, add almond flour, cocoa powder, sweetener, baking powder, salt and mix egg, vanilla extract and melted butter to make dough.
2. Make a circle with dough and put in pie plate, press sides and make fine edges.
3. Bake in preheated oven at 300F for 30 minutes and then let it cool.
4. Cream cheese frosting: in a bowl have cheese cream and beat well and add vanilla extract and more cream to make a fine and thick frosting.
5. Spread it on the chocolate crust evenly.
6. Toppings: decorate top with berries, microwave chocolate for topping and spread it on the crust top.
7. Put it in freezer for 20 minutes and serve.

Nutrition Information:
Calories: 473 kcal— Total Fat: 42g — Total Carbs: 3.1g— Protein: 19g

23. KETO MINI BLUEBERRY CHEESECAKES

- **For crust:**
-
- 1 cup almond flour
- 1 tbsp sweetener
- 2 tbsp coconut oil
- 1/4 tsp vanilla extract
- Pinch of salt

For cheesecake
- 8 oz cream cheese
- 1/2 cup sweetener

- 1 cup sour cream
- 1 tsp vanilla extract
- Blueberry topping
- 1 cup fresh blueberries
- 2 tbsp water
- 1/2 tbsp lemon juice
- 1/4 tsp xanthan gum

TOTAL TIME
38 MINUTES

DIRECTIONS

1. **For crust**: in a bowl mix almond flour, sweetener, coconut oil, vanilla extract and salt, stir well and make dough.
2. Take muffin cups and place dough evenly in cups.
3. Bake them for 8 minutes in a preheated oven at 325C until golden brown.
4.
5. **Cheesecake filling**: in a bowl have cream cheese and beat with electric beater, now add sweetener and beat until turn fluffy.
6. In a bowl mix sour cream and cheese cream mixture with vanilla extract and mix well. Now fill the crust with cheesecake filling and cool for an hour.
7. Blueberry sauce: in a pan put blueberries, water and lemon juice and cook on medium flam, now turn flam low and add xanthan gum and stir for 2 to 3 minutes.
8. After that remove it and let it cool.
9. Spread on muffins and garnish with berries and serve.

Nutrition Information:
Calories: 332 kcal— Total Fat: 32.3g — Total Carbs: 4.6g— Protein: 21g

24. PEANUT BUTTER PROTEIN BALLS

- **1 cup peanut butter**
- **2 tsp vanilla extract**
- **1/4 cup honey**
- **1 1/2 cup oats**
- **1/2 cup coconut**
- **A pinch of salt**
- **2-4 tsp water or use vanilla extract**
- **1/4 cup Chocolate chips**

TOTAL TIME
10 MINUTES

DIRECTIONS

1. Take a bowl, add peanut butter, honey and vanilla extract and mix well.
2. Now add oats, coconut, salt or chocolate chips and stir the mixture until it holds together.
3. To make a mixture use water or additional vanilla extract and make balls.
4. Let it rest at room temperature until combine and serve.

Nutrition Information:
Calories: 446 kcal— Total Fat: 42.8g — Total Carbs: 2.7g— Protein: 25.2g

25. FLUFFY LOW CARB KETO BLUEBERRY PANCAKES

INGREDIENTS

- 1/2 cup almond flour
- 1 tsp cinnamon
- 2 tbsp coconut flour
- 1/2 tsp baking powder
- 1-2 tbsp sweetener
- 3 eggs
- 1/4 cup almond milk
- 1/4 cup blueberries
-

TOTAL TIME
10 MINUTES

DIRECTIONS

1. In a bowl add almond flour, coconut flour, cinnamon, sweetener, baking powder, eggs and milk and blend all ingredients well until smooth.
2. Now pour blueberries in a mixture and stir well.
3. Let it set for 5 minutes.
4. Heat pan on medium flam and pour 1/4 cup of mixture and cook both sides until golden brown.
5. Prepare and serve immediately or for later.

Nutrition Information:
Calories: 446 kcal— Total Fat: 42.8g — Total Carbs: 2.7g— Protein: 25.2g

26. PALEO VEGAN CHOCOLATE COCONUT CRUNCH BAR

INGREDIENTS

- **1 1/2 cup chocolate chips**
- **1/2 cup sweetener**
- **1 cup peanut butter**
- **1/4 cup coconut oil**
- **1 1/2 cup shredded coconut**
- **1 1/2 cup nuts**

TOTAL TIME
10 MINUTES

DIRECTIONS

1. Take a microwave friendly bowl and add chocolate chips, peanut butter, sweetener and coconut oil and let it melt and combine.
2. Add coconut and nuts into mixture and whisk well.
3. Take a pan and place parchment paper in it.
4. Pour the mixture in pan and spread evenly. Refrigerate and serve.

Nutrition Information:
Calories: 667 kcal— Total Fat: 41.5g — Total Carbs: 6.4g— Protein: 49.9g

27. LOW CARB CARAMELS COCONUT

- **4 tbsp unsalted butter**
- **1 tsp erythritol sweetener**
- **4 tbsp heavy cream**
- **1 tsp salt**

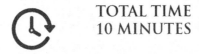

**TOTAL TIME
10 MINUTES**

DIRECTIONS

1. Take a pan and melt butter until turn golden brown.
2. Pour heavy cream in butter and heat at low flam for 1 minute.
3. Now add sweetener, pinch of salt and stir well.
4. Cook the mixture until it turns thick and sticky.
5. Pour the caramel into container and let it cool down.
6. Refrigerate it for later use or eat with dessert.

Nutrition Information:
Calories: 392 kcal— Total Fat: 35.5g — Total Carbs: 7.4g— Protein: 16.6g

28. HOMEMADE NUTELLA PIE

INGREDIENTS

- **25 Oreo cookies**
- **13 oz nutella**
- **5 tbsp melted butter**
- **8 oz cream cheese**
- **8 oz whipped topping**

**TOTAL TIME
25 MINUTES**

DIRECTIONS

1. Ground Oreo cookies and put them in a bowl.
2. Pour melted butter over cookie mixture and stir well.
3. Pour the mixture in a pan and press with a cup and place in freezer for 20 minutes.
4. Now pour some nutella over the pie crust and place in freezer again.
5. Take a bowl add cream cheese and remaining nutella and beat until creamy, mix with whipped topping and pour into the mixture and spread evenly.
6. Refrigerate for 2 hours before serving.

Nutrition Information:
Calories: 444 kcal— Total Fat: 52g — Total Carbs: 8.2g— Protein: 14.5g

29. KETO PANCAKES

- **2 eggs**
- **2 tsp erythritol**
- **2oz whipping cream**
- **Pinch salt**
- **2 oz almond flour**
- **1/4 tsp baking powder**
- **1 tsp unsalted butter**

**TOTAL TIME
8 MINUTES**

DIRECTIONS

1. Separate egg white and yolks. In a bowl add egg yolks, whipping cream, salt and mix until smooth.
2. In small bowl mix almond flour, baking powder and egg mixture and whisk well.
3. In a separate bowl beat egg whites with electric beater, now mix egg white foam with mixture evenly.
4. Heat a pan on medium flam and grease with butter, use spoon to pour mixture.
5. Cook each side for 2 minutes until turn brown.
6. Dish out and serve.

Nutrition Information:
Calories: 322 kcal— Total Fat: 29.9g — Total Carbs: 3.2g— Protein: 27.2g

30. LOW CARB KETO ITALIAN HOAGIE BISCUITS

INGREDIENTS

- **4 oz cream cheese**
- **1/4 cup heavy cream**
- **1 egg**
- **1/4 cup water**
- **1 packet Italian dressing**
- **1 1/4 cup almond flour**
- **1 cup provolone cheese**
- **1 cup chopped deli meat like pepperoni**

TOTAL TIME
35 MINUTES

DIRECTIONS

1. Take a blender adds cheese cream, egg, and water, heavy cream and Italian dressing mix and blend them well.
2. In a bowl add almond flour and prepared mixture and mix well.
3. Add chopped deli meat and cheese and combine.
4. Preheat oven at 350.
5. Take a baking muffin cups and grease with butter.
6. Fill almost 12 cups with the mixture and bake for 20 minutes.
7. Enjoy hot or chill.

Nutrition Information:
Calories: 223 kcal— Total Fat: 20g — Total Carbs: 10.2g— Protein: 15.5g

31. KETO CHOCOLATE MUFFINS

INGREDIENTS

- **1 cup almond flour**
- **1/2 cup erythritol**
- **1/2 cup coco powder**
- **1 1/2 tsp baking powder**
- **1 tsp vanilla extract**
- **2/3 cup heavy cream**
- **3 eggs**
- **3 oz butter**
- **1/2 cup sugar free chocolate chips**

TOTAL TIME
30 MINUTES

DIRECTIONS

1. Take a bowl add almond flour, coco powder, erythritol and baking powder, then add vanilla extract, eggs and heavy cream and mix well.
2. After that add butter and mix again, then add chocolate chips and stir.
3. Grease muffin cups and prepare 12 cups filled with mixture.
4. Bake into preheated oven 175C for 20 minutes.
5. Allow them to cool and serve.

Nutrition Information:
Calories: 244 kcal— Total Fat: 19g — Total Carbs: 4.2g— Protein: 5.5g

32. VIDALIA ONION SWISS DIP

INGREDIENTS

- **3 cup sweet onion chopped**
- **1 tsp pepper sauce**
- **2 cups Swiss cheese shredded**
- **Ground black pepper**
- **2 cups mayonnaise**
- **1/4 cup horseradish**

**TOTAL TIME
35 MINUTES**

DIRECTIONS

1. Take a bowl add sweet onion, horseradish, pepper sauce, mayonnaise and Swiss cheese, mix them well and transfer into pie plate.
2. Preheat oven at 375.
3. Now put the plate into oven and bake for 25 to 30 minutes until edges turn golden brown.
4. Sprinkle pepper to taste and serve with crackers.

Nutrition Information:
Calories: 294 kcal— Total Fat: 25g — Total Carbs: 12g— Protein: 7.2g

33. ROASTED PARMESAN CARROTS

INGREDIENTS

- **1lb peeled carrots**
- **1/4 tsp dried thyme**
- **1 tsp olive oil**
- **1/2 tsp salt**
- **1/4 tsp pepper**

TOTAL TIME
30 MINUTES

DIRECTIONS

1. Cut the carrots in half and small stick shape slices.
2. Take a baking pan adds carrots, olive oil, salt, pepper and thyme and mix it well and spread in pan evenly.
3. Preheat oven at 450, roast the mixture in oven for 12 to 15 minutes, after that serve with sauce or cheese.

Nutrition Information:
Calories: 204 kcal— Total Fat: 11g — Total Carbs: 4.2g— Protein: 1.5g

34. CILANTRO LIME SHRIMP

- **2 tbsp olive oil**
- **Black pepper to taste**
- **4 garlic cloves**
- **1lb shrimp peeled**
- **2 limes for juice**
- **3 tbsp unsalted butter**
- **1/4 tsp salt**
- **1/2 cup chopped cilantro**

TOTAL TIME
10 MINUTES

DIRECTIONS

1. Take a large skillet and add olive oil, garlic and sauté for 1 minute on medium flame.
2. After that add 1 tsp salt, 1/2 tsp black pepper and 1lb peeled shrimp or cook for 2 minutes until it turn pink.
3. Turn off the flame and add butter and cilantro, mix well until butter completely melts and dissolve and serve.

Nutrition Information:
Calories: 274 kcal— Total Fat: 19g — Total Carbs: 3.2g— Protein: 19.5g

35. PARMESAN ROASTED BROCCOLI

INGREDIENTS

- **4 to 5 pound broccoli**
- **1/2 tsp black pepper**
- **4 garlic cloves**
- **2 tsp lemon juice**
- **Olive oil**
- **3tbsp pine nuts**
- **1 1/2 tsp salt**
- **1/3 cup fresh parmesan cheese**
- **12 fresh basil leaves**

**TOTAL TIME
35 MINUTES**

DIRECTIONS

1. Preheat oven at 425F.
2. Cut the broccoli with florets and place it on a large pan sheet.
3. Add garlic and olive oil on broccoli and toss them well. Sprinkle salt and black pepper and roast them in oven for at least 20 to 25 minutes.
4. After that remove it from oven add 1tbsp olive oil and lemon juice, pine nuts, parmesan cheese and basil, mix it well and serve.

Nutrition Information:
Calories: 592 kcal— Total Fat: 53.9g — Total Carbs: 1.3g— Protein: 26.4g

36. SAUSAGE COBB SALAD LETTUCE WRAPS

INGREDIENTS

- 1/3 cup blue cheese, grated
- 4 eggs, cooked and minced
- 6 lettuce leaves
- 1 pound sausage
- 2 tablespoons chives, fresh chopped
- ¼ cup watercress, minced
- 1 tomato, minced
- 1 avocado, peeled and cubed
- ¾ cup salad dressing

TOTAL TIME
25 MINUTES

DIRECTIONS

1. In a bowl mix the cheese, watercress, and dressing.
2. In a pan, over the medium flame cook the sausage for 7 to 8 minutes and mix it in chives.
3. Set lettuce leaves in a plate and spoons the mixtures on it and on its top add eggs, tomato, avocado, and dressing mixture.

Nutrition Information:
Calories: 592 kcal — Total Fat: 29g — Total Carbs: 53g — Protein: 2.5g

37. MEXICAN CABBAGE ROLL SOUP

INGREDIENTS

- **1 pound beef, thin sliced**
- **12 ounces green chilies, mined**
- **6 cups cabbage, chopped**
- **½ teaspoon salt**
- **1 onion, minced**
- **1 tablespoon olive oil**
- **¼ teaspoon black pepper**
- **¾ teaspoon garlic powder**
- **1 can beef broth**
- **2 tablespoons cilantro, chopped**
- **2 cups of water**
-

**TOTAL TIME
45 MINUTES**

DIRECTIONS

1. In a pan cook beef in oil for 7 minutes on a medium-high flame and remove it in a plate.
2. In the same pan add onion and cabbage and cook for 6 minutes.
3. Add beef and other remaining ingredients in it and cook it for 10 minutes in a covered pan over the low flame and its ready to serve.

Nutrition Information:
Calories: 464 kcal— Total Fat: 65.5g — Total Carbs: 1.5g— Protein: 13.5g

38. LEMON ALMOND COCONUT CAKE

INGREDIENTS

- **250g almond**
- **60g desiccated coconut**
- **Pinch of salt**
- **150g natural sugar**
- **1 teaspoon vanilla extract**
- **zest of 1 large lemon**
- **3 eggs**
- **200g butter, melted**

- **Handful of almond flakes**

**TOTAL TIME
50 MINUTES**

DIRECTIONS

1. Preheat oven to 180°C.
2. Grease and line around cake tin with baking paper.
3. In medium bowl take almond, coconut, salt, and sugar, vanilla and lemon zest.
4. Add eggs and cooled butter to the dry mixture.
5. Mix the cake batter until smooth and thoroughly mixed.
6. Put the mixture in prepared cake tin.
7. Scatter with almond flakes.
8. Bake for approximately 40-45 minutes until lightly browned and cooked through the middle. Remove from oven and cool for 15-20 minutes and serve!

Nutrition Information:
Calories: 592 kcal— Total Fat: 53g — Total Carbs: 29g— Protein: 25g

39. PEANUT BUTTER & JAM CUPS

- ¼ **cup water**
- **1 teaspoon grass-fed gelatin**
- ¾ **cup coconut oil**
- ¾ **cup raspberries**
- **6 to 8 tablespoon Stevia**
- ¾ **cup peanut butter**

TOTAL TIME
45 MINUTES

DIRECTIONS

1. Line a muffin pan with parchment paper.
2. In a pan, combine the raspberries and water over medium heat. Bring to a boil and then reduce the heat and let the water dry.
3. Mash the berries with a fork.
4. Add in 2 to 4 tablespoon of the powdered sweetener.
5. Add in the grass fed gelatin and set aside to cool.
6. Now make peanut butter mixture.
7. In pan put the peanut butter and coconut oil.
8. Cook for 30 to 60 seconds, until melted.
9. Also add in 2 to 4 tablespoon of the powdered sweetener.
10. Put half of the peanut butter mixture in muffin pan and put in the freezer to firm up, about 15 minutes.
11. Divide the raspberry mixture among the muffin cups and top with the remaining peanut butter mixture.
12. Refrigerate until firm.

Nutrition Information:
Calories: 594 kcal— Total Fat: 53g — Total Carbs: 28g— Protein: 27g

40. KETO PUMPKIN PIE

Crust:
- 2 2/3 cup almond flour
- 3 eggs
- 6 tbsp unsalted butter
- 6 tbsp swerve
- 1 tsp salt

Filling:
- 15 oz pumpkin puree
- 1/2 cup heavy cream
- 2 eggs

- 1 cup swerve
- 1 tbsp pumpkin pie spice
- 1 tsp vanilla extract
- 1 tsp maple flavoring

TOTAL TIME
65 MINUTES

DIRECTIONS

1. Crust: in a bowl mix all ingredients and make smooth dough.
2. Preheat oven at 325F, take pie pan and grease its base. Set dough in pan and bake for 12-15 minutes.
3. Filling: in bowl add pumpkin puree, heavy cream, eggs, swerve, pumpkin pie spice, vanilla extract and maple flavoring and combine them well.
4. Pour the mixture on pie crust and cover its edges.
5. Bake it for 30-40 minutes.
6. Let it cool and serve.

Nutrition Information:
Calories: 492 kcal— Total Fat: 50g — Total Carbs: 39g— Protein: 22g

41. CINNAMON SUGAR DONUTS WITH ALMOND FLOUR

INGREDIENTS

- 1/2 cup almond flour
- 1 tsp cinnamon
- 1/3 cup erythritol
- 1/8 tsp salt
- 1/4 cup butter
- 1/4 cup almond milk
- 2 eggs
- 1/2 tsp vanilla extract

- **Coating:**
- 1 tsp cinnamon
- 3 tbsp butter

**TOTAL TIME
40 MINUTES**

DIRECTIONS

1. Take a bowl and mix almond flour, erythritol, baking powder, cinnamon and salt.
2. In bowl whisk butter, almond milk, egg, vanilla extracts and combines with dry ingredients.
3. Take donut baking try and pour mixture into it evenly.
4. Bake it for 22-25 minutes on preheated oven at 177C until golden brown.
5. In a bowl prepare cinnamon coating by mixing butter with cinnamon.
6. When donuts are cool down apply butter with brush and roll in coating.

Nutrition Information:
Calories: 298 kcal— Total Fat: 18.7g — Total Carbs: 10.8g— Protein: 22.6g

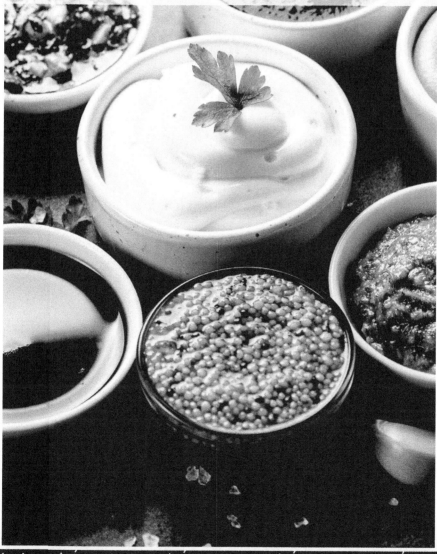

CHAPTER 10: SAUCES & DRESSINGS RECIPES

1. CRANBERRY SAUCE

INGREDIENTS

- **2½ teaspoons orange zest**
- **12 ounces cranberries**
- **¼ cup orange juice**
- **2 tablespoons maple syrup**
- **Salt**
- **1 cup sugar**

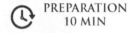 **PREPARATION
10 MIN**

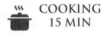 **COOKING
15 MIN**

 **SERVES
4**

DIRECTIONS

1. In the Instant Pot, mix the orange juice with maple syrup and stir well.
2. Add the orange zest and almost all of the cranberries, stir, cover and cook on the
3. Manual setting for 2 minutes. Release the pressure, uncover the Instant Pot, and set it on Sauté mode.
4. Add the rest of the cranberries, a pinch of salt, and the sugar, stir and cook until sugar dissolves.
5. Serve chilled.

Nutrition Value: Calories: 151 Fat: 0.4 Fiber: 1 Carbs: 39 Protein: 0.4

2. SIMPLE SPAGHETTI SAUCE

INGREDIENTS

- 1 and ⅔ pounds beef, ground
- 2 carrots, peeled and chopped
- 4 garlic cloves, peeled and minced
- 2 celery ribs, chopped
- 28 ounces canned crushed tomatoes
- 1 yellow onion, peeled and chopped
- 2 bay leaves
- 1 tablespoon olive oil
- Dried basil
- Dried oregano
- Red wine
- Salt and ground black pepper, to taste

For the chicken stock mix:
- 1 cup chicken stock
- 2 tablespoons soy sauce
- 3 tablespoons tomato paste
- 2 tablespoons fish sauce
- 1 tablespoon Worcestershire sauce

 PREPARATION 10 MIN

 COOKING 40 MIN

 SERVES 6

DIRECTIONS

1. Set the Instant Pot on Sauté mode, add the beef, salt, pepper, and oil, stir and brown for 7 minutes.
2. Transfer the beef to a bowl when it's brown and set it aside for now.
3. In a bowl, mix the stock with the fish sauce, soy sauce, tomato paste, and Worcestershire sauce and stir well.
4. Heat up you Instant Pot again, add the onions, garlic, bay leaves, basil, and oregano, stir and cook for 5 minutes.
5. Add the celery, carrots, salt, and pepper, stir and cook for 3 minutes.
6. Add the wine, chicken stock, beef, and crushed tomatoes on top. Cover the Instant Pot and cook on the Manual setting for 10 minutes.
7. Release the pressure, uncover the Instant Pot, add more salt and pepper, if needed, set the Instant Pot on Manual mode and cook the sauce for 4 minutes.
8. Serve with your favorite pasta.

Nutrition Value: Calories: 281 Fat: 16 Fiber: 5 Carbs: 20 Protein: 17

3. MARINARA SAUCE

INGREDIENTS

- **56 ounces canned crushed tomatoes**
- **3 garlic cloves, peeled and minced**
- **½ cup red lentils**
- **1 cup sweet potato, diced**
- **Salt and ground black pepper, to taste**
- **1½ cups water**

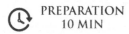 PREPARATION
10 MIN

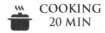 COOKING
20 MIN

 SERVES
8

DIRECTIONS

1. Set the Instant Pot on Sauté mode, add the lentils, sweet potatoes, salt, pepper, and garlic, stir and cook them for 2 minutes.
2. Add the water and tomatoes, stir, cover the Instant Pot and cook on the Manual setting for 13 minutes.
3. Release the pressure, uncover the Instant Pot, puree everything using an immersion blender.
4. Add more salt and pepper, if needed, set the Instant Pot on Manual mode, and cook the sauce for 4 minutes.

Nutrition Value: Calories: 60 Fat: 2 Fiber: 2 Carbs: 9 Protein: 2

4. ANCHO CHILI SAUCE

INGREDIENTS

- **5 ancho chilies, dried, seedless and chopped**
- **2 garlic cloves, peeled and crushed**
- **Salt and ground black pepper, to taste**
- **1½ cups water**
- **1½ teaspoons sugar**
- **½ teaspoon dried oregano**
- **½ teaspoon cumin**
- **2 tablespoons apple cider vinegar**

 PREPARATION 10 MIN   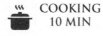 **COOKING 10 MIN**   **SERVES 8**

DIRECTIONS

1. In the Instant Pot mix the water chilies, garlic, salt, pepper, sugar, cumin, and oregano, stir, cover and cook on the Manual setting for 8 minutes.
2. Release the pressure for 5 minutes, uncover the Instant Pot, and pour sauce into a blender.
3. Add the vinegar, blend well and transfer everything to a bowl.

Nutrition Value: Calories: 50 Fat: 2 Fiber: 0 Carbs: 2

5. ZUCCHINI PESTO

- **1 yellow onion, peeled and chopped**
- **1 tablespoon extra virgin olive oil**
- **1½ pounds zucchini, chopped**
- **Salt, to taste**
- **½ cup water**
- **1 bunch fresh basil, chopped**

- **2 garlic cloves, peeled and minced**

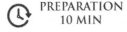 **PREPARATION**
10 MIN

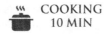 **COOKING**
10 MIN

 SERVES
4

DIRECTIONS

1. Set the Instant Pot on Sauté mode, add the oil and heat it up.
2. Add the onion, stir and cook 4 minutes.
3. Add the zucchini, salt and water, stir, cover, and cook on the Manual setting for 3 minutes.
4. Release the pressure, uncover the Instant Pot, add the garlic and basil and blend everything using an immersion blender.
5. Transfer to a bowl, and serve.

Nutrition Value: Calories: 71 Fat: 5 Fiber: 2.3 Carbs: 2 Protein: 1.

6. VEGETARIAN SAUCE

INGREDIENTS

- **1 yellow onion, peeled and chopped**
- **2 tablespoons olive oil**
- **5 celery ribs**
- **8 carrots, peeled and chopped**
- **4 beets, peeled and chopped**
- **1 butternut squash, peeled and chopped**
- **8 garlic cloves, peeled and minced**
- **1 cup vegetable stock**
- **¼ cup lemon juice**
- **1 bunch fresh basil, chopped**
- **2 bay leaves**
- **Salt and ground black pepper, to taste**

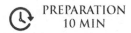 **PREPARATION 10 MIN**   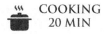 **COOKING 20 MIN**   **SERVES 8**

DIRECTIONS

1. Set the Instant Pot on Sauté mode, add the oil and heat it up.
2. Add the celery, onion, and carrots, stir and cook for 4 minutes.
3. Add the beets, squash, garlic, stock, lemon juice, basil, bay leaves, salt, and pepper, stir, cover and cook for 12 minutes at Manual.
4. Release the pressure, uncover the Instant Pot, discard the bay leaves, puree sauce using an immersion blender, transfer to a bowl, and serve.

Nutrition Value: Calories: 79 Fat: 1 Fiber: 0.4 Carbs: 5 Protein: 3

7. BARBECUE SAUCE

INGREDIENTS

- 1 tablespoon sesame seed oil
- ½ cup tomato puree
- 1 yellow onion, peeled and chopped
- ½ cup water
- 4 tablespoons white wine vinegar
- 4 tablespoons honey
- 1 teaspoon salt

- ½ teaspoon garlic powder
- 1 teaspoon liquid smoke
- 1 teaspoon Tabasco sauce
- 1/8 teaspoon cumin
- 1/8 teaspoon ground cloves
- 5 ounces dried seedless plums

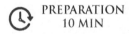 PREPARATION
10 MIN

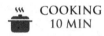 COOKING
10 MIN

 SERVES
8

DIRECTIONS

1. Set the Instant Pot on Sauté mode, add the oil and heat it up.
2. Add the onion, stir and cook for 5 minutes.
3. Add the tomato puree, honey, water, vinegar, salt, garlic, Tabasco sauce, liquid smoke, cumin, and cloves and stir everything very well.
4. Add the plums and stir well. Cover the Instant Pot and cook on the Manual setting for 10 minutes.
5. Release the pressure, uncover the Instant Pot, blend everything with an immersion blender, transfer sauce to a bowl, and serve.

Nutrition Value: Calories: 20 Fat: 0.4 Fiber: 0.4 Carbs: 3.5 Protein: 0.1

8. GRAVY

INGREDIENTS

- **Turkey neck, gizzard, livers, and heart**
- **1 tablespoon vegetable oil**
- **½ cup dry vermouth**
- **1 yellow onion, peeled and chopped**
- **1 quart turkey stock**
- **1 bay leaf**
- **4 tablespoons butter**
- **2 thyme sprigs**
- **4 tablespoons white flour**
- **Salt and ground black pepper, to taste**

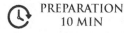 **PREPARATION**
10 MIN

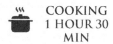 **COOKING**
1 HOUR 30 MIN

 SERVES
2

DIRECTIONS

1. Set the Instant Pot on Sauté mode, add the oil and heat it up.
2. Add the turkey pieces and onion, stir and cook for 3 minutes.
3. Stir again and cook for 3 minutes.
4. Add the vermouth, stock, bay leaf, and thyme and stir.
5. Cover the Instant Pot and cook on the Manual setting for 36 minutes.
6. Release the pressure for 20 minutes, strain the stock, reserve the turkey giblets and let them cool down, remove gristle and dice them into small pieces.
7. Heat up a pan with the butter over medium heat, add the flour, stir, and cook for 3 minutes.
8. Add the strained stock, stir well, increase heat to medium high and simmer for 20 minutes, stirring frequently.
9. Add salt, pepper, and the giblets, stir well, and serve.

Nutrition Value: Calories: 181 Fat: 10 Fiber: 1 Carbs: 11.4 Protein: 10.5

9. CHEESE SAUCE

INGREDIENTS

- **2 cups processed cheese, cut into chunks**
- **1 cup Italian sausage, cooked and chopped**
- **5 ounces canned tomatoes and green chilies, diced**
- **4 tablespoons water**

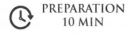 PREPARATION
10 MIN

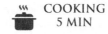 COOKING
5 MIN

 SERVES
4

DIRECTIONS

1. In the Instant Pot, mix sausage with cheese, tomatoes, and chilies and water.
2. Stir, cover and cook on the Manual setting for 5 minutes.
3. Release the pressure, uncover the Instant Pot, transfer sauce to a bowl, and serve with your favorite pasta or vegetables.

Nutrition Value: Calories: 110 Fat: 8.5 Fiber: 0.4 Carbs: 4.3 Protein: 4.32

10. MUSHROOM SAUCE

INGREDIENTS

- 1 yellow onion, peeled and chopped
- ¼ cup olive oil
- 1 tablespoon flour
- Salt and ground black pepper, to taste
- 1 tablespoon thyme, chopped
- 3 garlic cloves, peeled and minced
- 1¼ cup chicken stock
- ¼ cup dry sherry
- 10 ounces shiitake mushrooms, chopped
- 10 ounces cremini mushrooms, chopped
- 10 ounces button mushrooms, chopped
- 1-ounce Parmesan cheese, grated
- ½ cup heavy cream
- 1 tablespoons parsley, diced

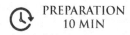 **PREPARATION** 10 MIN 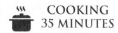 **COOKING** 35 MINUTES   **SERVES** 6

DIRECTIONS

1. Set the Instant Pot on Sauté mode, add the oil and heat it up.
2. Add the onion, salt, and pepper, stir and cook for 5 minutes.
3. Add the garlic, flour, and thyme, stir and cook for 1 minute.
4. Add sherry, stock, and the mushrooms, stir, cover, and cook on the Manual setting for 25 minutes.
5. Release pressure, uncover the Instant Pot, add the cream, cheese, and parsley, stir, and set the Instant Pot on Manual mode.
6. Cook for 5 minutes, transfer to a bowl, and serve.

Nutrition Value: Calories: 140 Fat: 5.7 Fiber: 3.1 Carbs: 13 Protein: 7.4

11. HOT SAUCE

INGREDIENTS

- **12 ounces hot peppers, chopped**
- **2 teaspoons salt**
- **1¼ cups apple cider vinegar**

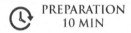 PREPARATION
10 MIN

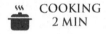 COOKING
2 MIN

 SERVES
6

DIRECTIONS

1. Put peppers into the Instant Pot.
2. Add the vinegar and salt, stir, cover, and cook on the Manual setting for 2 minutes.
3. Release the pressure for 15 minutes, uncover the Instant Pot, and puree everything using your immersion blender.
4. Transfer to jars, and serve when needed.

Nutrition Value: Calories: 12 Fat: 0.04 Fiber: 0 Carbs: 0.04 Protein: 0.06

12. STRAWBERRY SAUCE

- **1 ounce orange juice**
- **⅛ cup sugar**
- **1 pound strawberries, cored and cut into halves**
- **Ground ginger**
- **½ teaspoon vanilla extract**

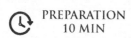 PREPARATION
10 MIN

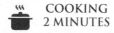 COOKING
2 MINUTES

 SERVES
8

DIRECTIONS

1. In the Instant Pot, mix the strawberries with sugar, stir, and leave them aside for 10 minutes.
2. Add the orange juice, stir, cover, and cook on the Manual setting for 2 minutes.
3. Release the pressure for 15 minutes, uncover the Instant Pot, add the vanilla extract, and ginger, puree using an immersion blender and refrigerate until ready for use.

Nutrition Value: Calories: 60 Fat: 0 Carbs: 13 Protein: 1

13. CAULIFLOWER SAUCE

INGREDIENTS

- **2 tablespoons butter**
- **8 garlic peeled and cloves, minced**
- **7 cups vegetable stock**
- **6 cups cauliflower florets**
- **Salt and ground black pepper, to taste**
- **½ cup milk**

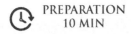 PREPARATION
10 MIN

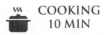 COOKING
10 MIN

 SERVES
6

DIRECTIONS

1. Set the Instant Pot on Sauté mode, add the butter and melt it.
2. Add garlic, salt, and pepper, stir, cook for 5 minutes and transfer to a bowl.
3. Add the stock and cauliflower to the Instant Pot, heat up, cover, and cook on the Manual setting for 7 minutes.
4. Release the pressure, transfer the cauliflower and 1 cup stock to your blender, add the salt, pepper, milk, and garlic and puree for a few minutes. Serve with pasta.

Nutrition Value: Calories: 119 Fat: 5 Fiber: 1 Carbs: 10 Protein: 8

14. MANGO SAUCE

INGREDIENTS

- 1 shallot, peeled and chopped
- 1 tablespoon vegetable oil
- ¼ teaspoon cardamom
- 2 tablespoons ginger, minced
- ½ teaspoon ground cinnamon
- 2 mangos, chopped
- 2 red hot chilies, chopped
- 1 apple, cored and chopped
- 2 teaspoons salt
- ¼ cup raisins
- 1¼ cup raw sugar
- 1¼ apple cider vinegar

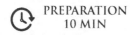 PREPARATION 10 MIN

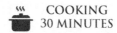 COOKING 30 MINUTES

 SERVES 4

DIRECTIONS

1. Set the Instant Pot on Sauté mode, add the oil and heat it up. Add the ginger and shallot, stir and cook for 5 minutes.
2. Add the cinnamon, hot peppers, and cardamom, stir and cook for 2 minutes.
3. Add the mangos, apple, raisins, sugar, and cider, stir and cook until the sugar melts.
4. Cover the Instant Pot and cook on the Manual setting for 7 minutes.
5. Release the pressure, uncover the Instant Pot, transfer to a pan, and simmer on medium heat for 15 minutes, stirring occasionally.
6. Transfer to jars, and serve when needed.

Nutrition Value: Calories: 80 Fat: 0.3 Fiber: 1 Carbs: 9 Protein: 0.9

15. TOMATO CHUTNEY

- **3 pounds tomatoes, cored, peeled, and chopped**
- **1 cup red wine vinegar**
- **1¾ cups sugar**
- **1-inch ginger piece, peeled and grated**
- **3 garlic cloves, peeled and minced**
- **2 onions, peeled and chopped**

- **¼ cup raisins**
- **¾ teaspoon ground cinnamon**
- **¼ teaspoon ground cloves**
- **½ teaspoon coriander**
- **¼ teaspoon nutmeg**
- **¼ teaspoon ground ginger**
- **Paprika**
- **1 teaspoon chili powder**

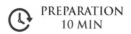 **PREPARATION**
10 MIN

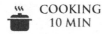 **COOKING**
10 MIN

 SERVES
6

DIRECTIONS

1. Mix the tomatoes and the grated ginger into the blender, pulse well, and transfer to the Instant Pot.
2. Add the vinegar, sugar, garlic, onions, raisins, cinnamon, cloves, coriander, nutmeg, ground ginger, paprika, and chili powder, stir, cover, and cook on the
3. Manual setting for 10 minutes.
4. Release the pressure, uncover the Instant Pot, transfer to jars, and serve when needed.

Nutrition Value: Calories: 140 Fat: 10 Fiber: 0 Carbs: 10 Protein: 4

16. TOMATO SAUCE

INGREDIENTS

- **2 pounds tomatoes, cored, peeled, and chopped**
- **1 apple, cored and chopped**
- **1 yellow onion, peeled and chopped**
- **6 ounces raisins, chopped**
- **3 ounces dates,**
- **chopped**
- **Salt, to taste**
- **3 teaspoons allspice**
- **½ pint vinegar**
- **½ pound brown sugar**

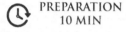 PREPARATION
10 MIN

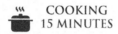 COOKING
15 MINUTES

 SERVES
20

DIRECTIONS

1. Put the tomatoes into the Instant Pot.
2. Add the apple, onion, raisins, dates, salt, allspice, and half of the vinegar, stir, cover, and cook on the Manual setting for 10 minutes.
3. Release the pressure, uncover the Instant Pot, set it on Manual mode, add the rest of the vinegar and sugar, stir, and simmer until the sugar dissolves.
4. Transfer to jars, and serve when needed.

Nutrition Value: Calories: 70 Fat: 4 Fiber: 1 Carbs: 8 Protein: 1.7

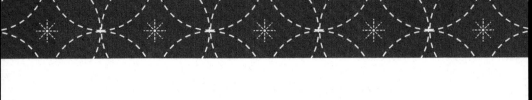

CHAPTER 11: KETO HEALTHY LIFESTYLE TO LOSE WEIGHT

The correct calorie and macronutrient intake effects the most important role in achieving high level physique goals. Tracking our total food intake is the easiest and most reliable way to lose body fat or gain lean body mass

The main purpose behind guide is to help you better understand the relationship between how much and what we eat and the way our bodies look. My hope is that this information will save you a lot of time and effort as well.

What Is Weight Loss

Weight loss is basically weight that you lose when your body undergoes a process of what the experts term as caloric deficiency. This can be achieved either by boosting your calories requirement through building of muscle mass whilst keeping your intake constant, or via calories restriction in the form of a diet where your daily calories intake is designed to be lesser than your daily requirement.

When your body finds itself in a state where calories input are lesser than what it needs for daily function, it will seek to get energy from stores of energy within your body. Most of the time these would be from the stores of glucose found in the liver as well as from your muscle. The other major energy store found in our body would be the fats that we carry on our frame. This is where the tricky part comes in. If your body isn't conditioned for burning fats, it will quickly use up the glucose stores and that is when the feeling of hunger will come in to potentially derail you from your weight loss mission.

Some Common Weight Loss Principles to Note

To help with the process of losing the unwelcome weight from your body, here are some of the more common principles which are good to base your weight loss strategies on.

Keep hunger at bay – Many folks start off on dieting to lose their excess weight and attempt to get healthy but quite a number fail and fall by the wayside. In the end, these folks have to resort to medications and drugs in order to suppress the symptoms and conditions that accompany obesity. It is definitely not a pretty sight, and it sometimes is quite depressing to see people consign themselves to such a fate when more efficient and healthier solutions are actually just around the corner.

They may have started off strong and seen results after some time, but invariably, the one thing that always put paid to these efforts would be the feeling of hunger that many of these diets entail. Take a plain calorie restriction diet plan for example, if your daily requirement works out to be about 1,750 calories, just polishing off a bagel for a snack would set you back by 250 calories. That is like one seventh of your total requirement. Imagine eating seven bagels for the whole day, would that be enough?

The trick of course is to get onto a diet and lifestyle change where you are able to feel full and keep the hunger pangs at bay and yet get your body to lose weight. Know of any diet that does just that?

Be sustainable – There are many ways to lose weight, that is for sure. Getting on the latest fad diet, juicing, fasting, going the vegan way. I have to say as a matter of fact that I hold all these methodologies in high esteem and it is my opinion that each one of them has their benefits for the human body.

Fasting for example, is a good way to let the body rebalance itself and to get rid of toxins that have built up over time. One of the side effects of fasting would be loss of body weight. However, you would not expect a person to fast for a lifetime, without any consumption of food. For any method of efficient weight loss, it must be sustainable in practice to allow for continued shedding of the excess pounds and also to prevent the dreaded bounce back in weight that has plagued so many

One of the benchmarks of sustainability for diets would be the ease of implementing it in everyday life. Imagine if you are on a diet that requires you to eat six to seven small meals a day, you would definitely have to pack for those meals and also find the time to consume them during the work day.

Exercise – Regarded as one of the main pillars for weight loss, exercise, especially strength training, can help to build muscles that burn more calories, not to mention getting you that ripped figure. Yes, it was always good to dream that there was some magic pill in the market that could get you whipped in shape without any effort, but alas, it still remains a dream.

Strength training, done through weights at home or by hitting the gym is one of the surest ways that weight can be lost. Most of the time, it would be advisable to have a schedule for the days that you work out to concentrate on specific muscle groups. This targeted training helps to speed muscle development, leading to higher calorie usage and hence weight loss.

There will be loads of resources online on how to work out a proper strength training routine. The more important thing is to have the discipline to keep plugging at it until you see or feel the results. Believe me, it will be worth it.

First of all, you have to take a look at your diet, the amount of exercise you get per week, how much sleep you get a night, and then use this information to understand how much it will have to change based on your goals.

If you're eating bad every day, going too fast food spots, and only feel your blood pumping when your favorite TV show is about to come on, and you're only sleeping five or six hours a night, of course, you are gonna feel bad, and look bad.

Don't worry because you are going to be learning all the process and you are going to be and feel healthier than ever.

You cannot expect your body to be able to look and feel its best when you don't give it the vitamins and nutrients it needs to be vigorous, healthy and attractive looking. There's no magic pill that you can take or some machine that you can put minimal effort into and expect to have abs by dinner time. It takes hard work, and consistency to tell your body it's going to change.

The great thing is your body wants to change; it wants to be healthy, it wants to be free of disease and sickness, it wants you to be proud and able to show it off, you just need to start the process by changing your diet and workout, (or adding an exercise).

Everybody has abs. Some people have long torsos and have six abs; some people have four, some even have eight. We all have them, but not everybody is comfortable proclaiming they have abs because they are covered by layers and layers of fat.

To strip the fat off, you need to expend (burn off/get rid of) more calories than you intake in a day.

It's not necessary to count calories though, and it's a lot simpler if we don't. All we need to do is

ating at regular times in the day, small healthy meals, and have some workout that we follow consistently three or more times a week.

Doing crunch after crunch will not make you get rid of the fat on your stomach. It might burn calories and strengthen your abdominals and make it so that when you are low enough body fat, they will be sharp and beautiful enough to be proud of really, but it's not as efficient as doing cardio, on the treadmill for example.

Don't worry; this is going to be fun! You are going to be healthy, with more energy, and a peaceful mind after reading this book. It is going to be tough, I know. But you are going to love the process, once you achieve your goals.

You are not alone. Many people are striving to be thinner, healthier and have a good quality of life. And many people do it... so I'm pretty sure you will.

Diet is a buzzword most people really don't want to hear. Diet supposedly means restriction; it means confining your life to salads and protein shakes. It makes people feel like they can't even have a life.

Don't believe them. In fact, we're going to change the meaning of the word "diet" right now. Diet simply means what you eat. When people say they're "going on a diet" they mean that they're going to buy in to some ridiculous fad that they will inevitably drop before the pounds even do. When I say the word diet, I just mean the content of what you use to feed yourself. What is your plate made up of? Nobody here is "going on a diet," I promise.

Now, let's talk about food and how we should eat it. First off, your diet is only one part of an overall lifestyle you need to be healthy. Instead of talking about the foods you can't have, I'm going to focus on the foods you should have more of.

Foods you should have more of:

This might be obvious to some. People tend to think they need to eat fruits and vegetables and not a lot more. You are wrong. It's more complicated than that. Here is what you should be eating to stay healthy and drop a little weight:

Green, leafy vegetables: sneak them into a smoothie or a flavorful salad. Keep the iceberg lettuce for the rabbits. You need spinach, kale, and arugula – a complex mix of leafy greens. My favorite thing to do is put them in a smoothie with some berries, bananas, or any fruits you enjoy. It's healthy, delicious, and you can't even taste the greens.

Complex Carbs:

Cutting carbs isn't always a great idea. It can leave you low on energy and craving high-carb, high-sugar foods later on. If you start your day with high fiber, complex carbs such as fruits, vegetables, oatmeal, whole grains, or bran cereal, you're far less likely to reach for the candy bar later.

Good Fats:

Fats, much like carbs, are foods we need in our diets. They help with brain function and heart health. They also keep you full longer and help to process vital nutrients. Good fats are found in foods such as avocados, olive oil, and nuts.

Do you see what we did here? I did not tell you what foods to cut, I told you what foods to add. As a result of adding those foods, you will automatically cut other, more harmful foods from your diet. Did you know that eating avocado or nuts can help curb chocolate cravings? That's because when you have a craving, it's your body's way of telling you what you need.

Besides these symptoms, you should also experience a whole host of beneficial symptoms. Some of the most beneficial symptoms, like an improvement in metabolism, and weight loss, will take longer to happen. But others happen within days. You will find your appetite begins to come under your control. As your insulin spikes and crashes disappear, your body gets used to having a steady supply of energy. This means that rather than feeling hungry every single time your blood sugar drops, and snacking between meals, you are eating a healthy meal and going straight through to the next one without feeling hungry.

You will find that yeast infections and skin conditions improve, or even disappear entirely. This is because your candida is not being fed, so it has nothing to grow from. Candida causes many types of yeast infection, and several types of skin problem, being the root cause of most cases of dandruff, for starters. It also makes other conditions, like eczema, worse, by irritating the skin and growing under and around dead skin cells.

You will find your moods are more even. That "hungry" feeling you get when your blood sugar drops is not normal. It is your body responding to a lack of glucose, trying to get you to eat carbs. At first you may feel the carb-hungry anger more intensely than usual, but after a couple of days your body gets used to not having those constant spikes and crashes in blood sugar. No energy crashes means no cravings, means no eating carbs, means no spikes, means no more crashes. It is vitally important to fight this cycle and restore order, even if you have no intention of following a ketogenic diet for life.

Low-Carb

The low-carbohydrate diet has been around since the beginning of human history. Pre-agricultural humans subsisted on what they could hunt or gather, which meant wild meat, game, fish, roots, berries, and other plant matter. Around 12,000 years ago, humans left their nomadic ways and began consuming more carbohydrates in the forms of cereal grains and legumes. Still, it was a far cry from today's endless supply of pasta and breadsticks.

Fast forward to the twentieth century when industrial food products, refined grains, and sugar became widely available and came with a side of obesity, heart disease, and diabetes. Instead of blaming refined carbs—which were novel foods in human evolution—people pointed the finger at fat.

Give Up Carbs, Not Flavor

To understand why a diet low in carbohydrates is so effective, it helps to have a basic scientific understanding of how and why our bodies use and store carbohydrates.

Whenever we eat foods containing carbohydrates, our blood sugar (also known as blood glucose) levels rise proportionate to the total amount of carbohydrates we have eaten (called the glycemic load) and how quickly that carbohydrate is absorbed (called the glycemic index). The pancreas, which is an organ that's located deep in the abdomen, releases the hormone insulin, which lowers blood glucose and makes it available to the cells.

When the body doesn't need glucose for immediate energy or to restore the energy stored in the muscles (called glycogen), the glucose is repackaged with fatty acids into more complex structures called triglycerides for long-term storage within the fat cells. If there isn't enough room in the existing fat cells, new fat cells are created, aided by insulin. Insulin also activates enzymes that increase fat storage and prevent fat from being used for fuel. Hence, when blood glucose levels and insulin production remain consistently high, fat storage is inevitable and fat metabolism (that is, the use of fat for fuel) cannot occur.

A low-carbohydrate, high-fat ketogenic diet keeps insulin levels low, which allows triglycerides to be broken down into fatty acids that can be burned as energy. Not only does this result in the loss of body fat, but it also ensures that a steady stream of energy is available to fuel your body. And it tastes pretty good, too!

Have You Met These Healthy Fats?

The ketogenic diet is necessarily high in fats. But not all fats are created equal. Partially hydrogenated oils contain trans fats (even when the package says "0 grams trans fat") and are found in margarine, peanut butter, and other processed foods. They are dangerous to your health because they increase inflammation and elevate LDL ("bad" cholesterol) and reduce HDL ("good" cholesterol), both of which increase the risk of heart disease and hinder weight loss. So just go with the real stuff. Here are my top five fats for a low-carb diet:

Avocados

Avocados are rich in monounsaturated fats, particularly oleic acid, which has been shown to decrease inflammation, lower the risk of heart disease, and improve insulin sensitivity. Monounsaturated fats are burned at a faster rate than other fats and increase metabolism. For example, a study published in 2013 found that the addition of half of an avocado with meals increased satiety for up to five hours following a meal among obese individuals. Avocados are also a great source of vitamin K, folate, vitamin C, potassium, and vitamin E. Potassium is especially important on a low-carb diet because it helps prevent muscle cramping, which can be a concern as you shed excess water weight.

Butter

It is no surprise that butter contributes flavor and a rich, velvety texture to foods, but you may be surprised to learn that butter, especially when it is sourced from organic, grass-fed cows, contains omega-3 fats, selenium, and vitamins A, D, E, and K. Butter has a low smoke point, so rather than using it for high-temperature cooking, use butter on cooked vegetables, in baking, or in quick, low-heat cooking methods, such as when making eggs. If you are sensitive to dairy proteins, try ghee (also called clarified butter), which has been heated and strained to remove the milk solids.

Coconut Oil

Coconut oil is the ketogenic dieter's best friend. It is a flavorful source of fatty acids that have been shown to correlate with increased calorie burning and weight loss. It is also easily converted into water-soluble molecules called ketone bodies in the liver, meaning you can get into ketosis more quickly by adding coconut oil to your diet (see "What Is Ketosis?" here). Coconut oil also increases metabolism while reducing appetite, so the calories you consume from coconut oil will be burned off and cause you to eat fewer other foods. It can be eaten raw in fat bombs (sweet or savory snack bites that provide nearly all of their calories from fat) or used for roasting, sautéing, or frying.

Extra-Virgin Olive Oil

Extra-virgin olive oil is rich in monounsaturated fats, contains antioxidants, is anti-inflammatory, may reduce the risk of heart disease, and ultimately can help you lose weight. For example, a study comparing the effects of a low-fat diet versus a diet enriched with extra-virgin olive oil found that women following a 1,500-calorie-a-day diet containing three tablespoons of olive oil lost twice as much weight as those consuming the same number of calories without the olive oil. For the greatest health benefits, use extra-virgin olive oil for low-heat cooking, in salad dressings, and to drizzle over cooked foods.

Nuts

Nuts such as walnuts, cashews, pistachios, almonds, and pecans contain monounsaturated and polyunsaturated fats, including omega-3 fatty acids, and can help reduce the risk of heart disease, lower diabetes risk, and encourage you to stick with your low-carb diet by improving satiety and ultimately helping you lose weight. Nuts contain about equal proportions of protein and carbohydrate, which is mostly in the form of fiber.

What Is Ketosis?

"Fat adaptation" is another term that describes ketosis. Being in ketosis naturally reduces your appetite. In fact, appetite reduction is one of the many appeals of fat adaptation because you can go for long stretches between meals—such as a busy day or a deliberate period of fasting— without feeling hungry or experiencing symptoms of low blood sugar.

In healthy people, nutritional ketosis is usually achieved within as few as three days of reducing daily carbohydrate intake to below 50 grams. However, people who are obese may have more difficulty achieving ketosis. Ketosis can also be induced by fasting, which counterintuitively may be easier for some people than eating a low-carb diet during the transition period. Always consult your physician before making any dietary changes.

A ketogenic diet may improve metabolic syndrome, insulin resistance, and type 2 diabetes. It is also used to treat people with epilepsy and other neurological disorders.

Going Keto

A ketogenic diet contains low carbohydrates, moderate protein, and high fat. The macronutrient composition of a ketogenic diet typically falls within the following ranges: 5 to 10 percent carbohydrates, 20 to 25 percent protein, and 70 percent fat. On a 2,000-calorie-per-day diet, that would look like 50 grams of carbohydrates, 100 grams of protein, and 155 grams of fat.

Some low-carbohydrate diets include very high levels of protein—as high as 50 percent of total calories. While protein promotes satiety, improves mood, and builds muscle, obtaining more than 30 percent of your calories from protein can have detrimental and even dangerous effects. Excess protein can be converted to glucose, which elevates insulin levels, hinders ketosis, and may stall weight loss. Worse yet, excess protein can cause kidney damage, weaken bones, and contribute to the growth of cancer cells.

Instead of replacing calories from carbohydrates with calories from protein, the ketogenic approach involves replacing those calories with calories from fat. Pairing a low-carbohydrate diet with a high-fat diet is essential to success because even during weight loss, your body can only burn a limited amount of stored body fat—about 69 calories per kilogram of nonessential body fat per day. You have to eat something to fuel your daily activity, and dietary fat is the best replacement for carbs. Dietary fat slows the release of glucose into the bloodstream and is satiating, so you won't feel hungry on a low-carb diet. Of course, always speak to your doctor before beginning any diet, especially if you have an existing medical condition.

Should You Count Calories?

While calories do matter even on a ketogenic diet, they don't necessarily need to be counted because ketosis results in a natural appetite reduction and reduced calorie intake. Nevertheless, calculating your basal metabolic rate (BMR) and total daily energy expenditure (TDEE) is useful for planning purposes and can be essential if you find that your weight loss has stalled on a low-carb diet.

CHAPTER 12: HOW TO PREVENT DIABETES WITH KETO DIET?

What is diabetes?

Diabetes includes disorders of blood sugar metabolism. In our society today, carbohydrates are the primary source of energy for the body.

To distribute the sugar in the body and into the cells, the pancreas produces the hormone insulin. Insulin docks on a cell to the insulin receptor, then lock open (GLUT-4), and glucose flows into the cell.

In diabetes, this mechanism is interrupted. For various reasons, no more sugar gets into the cell. Either because insulin no longer binds or Not enough sugar enters the cell (type 2 diabetes), or because the pancreas produces little or no insulin (type 1 diabetes), or because the complete Insulin pathway is interrupted at a certain point.

Type 1 diabetes

In type 1 diabetes, very little insulin is produced in the pancreas; here is an autoimmune disease. It destroys the immune system due to a malfunction of the pancreas, which then can no longer exercise his work.

Since insulin is no longer produced in some cases, but the sugar is needed in the cells, type 1 diabetes is insulin-dependent; In sensitive situations, extremely high blood sugar levels (700 mg/dl) and so-called ketoacidosis can occur.

Type 2 diabetes

Insulin is secreted in type 2 diabetes, but the pathway does not work to get the blood sugar into the cells. This is called insulin resistance or glucose intolerance. This form of diabetes is not always insulin-dependent, and the causes are manifold compared to type 1 diabetes.

It is also called the prosperity of diabetes. Until 100 years ago, this disease was practically only present in very rich sections of the population. Still, since the end of the Second World War, the incidence of this disease has increased dramatically - from all walks of life.

Both our medical system and the food and pharmaceutical industries seem to be overwhelmed by the problem of diabetes because prevalent treatment regimens tend not to improve the disease. Instead, there is always talk of "diabetes management."

Because of these facts and with some scientific studies behind us, we would like to propose today an alternative in diabetes: the ketogenic diet.

KETOGENIC NUTRITION IN DIABETES

Type 1 diabetes

There are no relevant clinical studies yet on which we can rely. Besides, type 1 diabetes is not as common as type 2 diabetes; not only are there more studies here, but also more testimonials.

Theoretically, the ketogenic diet should work well in type 1 diabetes.

Type 2 Diabetes

Ketogenic diets fit perfectly in type 2 diabetes.

A chronic disease of blood sugar metabolism meets a high-fat and low-carbohydrate diet, which causes a stable and low blood sugar levels and low insulin levels. And that fits perfectly, the studies show.

The problem is that with type 2 diabetes, the causes of the disease can be very diverse:

Became too much fast food eaten with highly processed foods, plenty of sugar, and trans fat?

Is there a lack of nutrients (e.g., chromium, magnesium, or vitamin A), which disturbs the energy transfer or the insulin pathway sensitively?

Is there obesity of metabolically active organs such as the pancreas or liver?

Is a strong overweight a chronically elevated blood lipid level, and thus a chronic inflammation and a disturbed blood sugar metabolism before?

Is there a genetic predisposition to the disease?

Is there a growth disorder on the pancreas (e.g., due to vitamin A deficiency), and is there only too little insulin produced?

Is there a chronic inflammation of the pancreas (pancreatitis), so that it comes only to a limited function?

Or: Is there a very inactive lifestyle in combination with other risk factors (obesity, fast food, smoking, loneliness)?

It becomes clear that the causes of diabetes can be diverse, but the following disease is more consistent in terms of symptoms. In order not only to "manage" diabetes but to treat it and reverse it, the cause of the disease must be addressed.

Type 2 diabetes and Ketogenic Diet

In the following diabetes risk factors, a well-formulated ketogenic diet, or at least a healthier lifestyle, can bring about a significant improvement: nutritional deficiency, pancreatitis, overweight, fast food, inactive lifestyle.

With these risk factors and causes, a healthy lifestyle is considered to be the basis of treatment. The ketogenic diet can make a valuable contribution here.

However, by far, the most common risk factor for diabetes is overweight: About 60% of all adults in Germany are overweight, overweight is a major cause of other diseases such as high blood pressure, insulin resistance (diabetes), abnormal blood lipid levels and cardiovascular disease. If obesity is reduced, diabetes improves in most cases.

We did not want to cause any confusion with the last chapter but point out the precarious situation, because to treat a disease, it is essential to know the causes. In most cases of diabetes, several of these risk factors are present at the same time - and in most cases of diabetes, a ketogenic diet can dramatically improve the disease

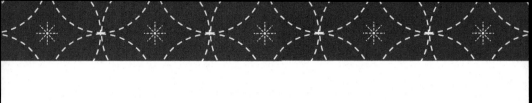

CONCLUSION

Now that you know that the Keto diet isn't as intimidating as you may have thought, the next step is to ditch the carbs, fill up on fatty foods and watch for the ketosis bliss to happen.

Remember, this diet is not one-size-fits-all type of diet, so don't expect your Keto journey to be like someone else's. The main point is for you to feel healthy, balanced, and beautiful in your own body. Do not push yourself too hard, and take the transformation one step at a time. If it all starts to get a bit too much for your taste, try the carb cycling and see if that will make a difference. Whatever you do, do it with caution and in moderation.

I promise, your healthy figure and balanced state of mind is waiting for you in ketosis. Purge the carbs and get there in under 2 weeks with the knowledge of this book.

Good luck and happy dieting!

93558887R00096